EAT RIGHT-
TO KEEP HEALTHY AND ENJOY LIFE MORE

Dr Denis Burkitt worked for nearly twenty years as a surgeon in a teaching hospital in East Africa. During this time he described a form of cancer which now bears his name (Burkitt's Lymphoma).

For this and other work he has received fellowships and awards from many countries. During the last ten years his studies into world-wide disease distribution related to diet have received international recognition. A Fellow of the Royal Society, he is a recent recipient of the Gold Medal of the British Medical Association.

Dr Burkitt has travelled extensively in all five continents lecturing and collecting information relevant to his research interests. He has co-edited *Treatment of Burkitt's Lymphoma* (1967), *Burkitt's Lymphoma* (1970) and *Refined Carbohydrate Foods and Disease* (1975).

Dr Burkitt values his home life far more than the recognition given his scientific work.

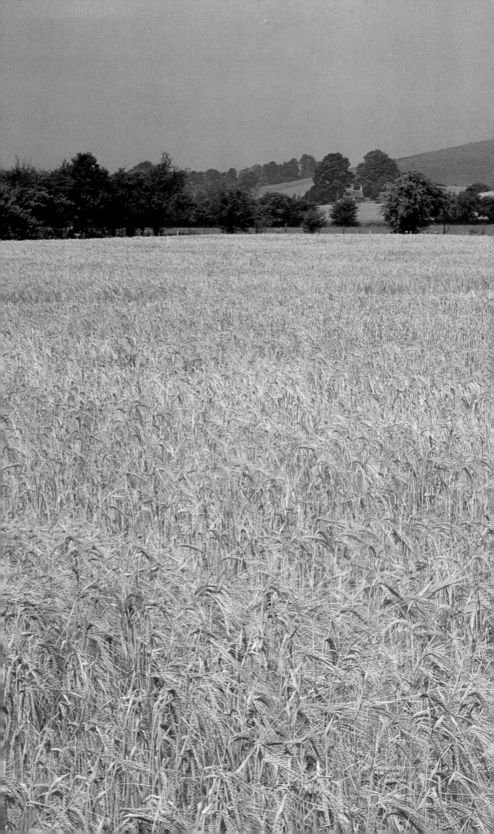

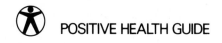
POSITIVE HEALTH GUIDE

EAT RIGHT-
TO KEEP HEALTHY AND ENJOY LIFE MORE
How simple diet changes can prevent many common diseases

Denis Burkitt

MD, FRCS, FRS

Arco Publishing, Inc.
New York

Published 1979 by Arco Publishing, Inc
219 Park Avenue South, New York,
N.Y. 1003

First published in the United Kingdom in
1979 by Martin Dunitz Limited

Cover and studio photographs by Rob
Matheson
Text filmset by Inforum Ltd, Portsmouth

**Library of Congress Cataloging in
Publication Data**

Burkitt, Denis Parsons.
Eat right — to keep healthy and enjoy life
more
   (Positive health guide)
   Bibliography: p. 1
   Includes index.
   1. Fiber deficiency diseases. 2. High-fiber
   diet. 3. Health. I. Title. II. Series.
RC627.F5B87   616.3'96   78–24492
ISBN 0–668–04676–7
ISBN 0–668–04682–1 pbk.

Printed in Hong Kong by
South China Printing Company Limited

CONTENTS

To Olive
Without her constant support, the writing of this book would not have been possible.

INTRODUCTION: THE REASON FOR FIBRE

In recent years doctors and the general public have become increasingly aware of the importance of diet in relation to health. As part of this awareness there has been a great surge of interest in the role of fibre or roughage in our food, and its possible protection against a large number of diseases which are very common in Western countries today.

Fibre is the part of food which is not digested. Whereas protein, fats and carbohydrates are almost entirely absorbed in the small intestine, fibre passes through to the large intestine virtually unchanged. Its value has been overlooked because it seemingly had little part to play nutritionally.

Nutrition is derived from the proteins, fats and carbohydrates in the foods we eat. The protein foods are mainly meat, fish, dairy produce, nuts, flour and other cereals. Fats come from butter, vegetable oils, margarine, as well as from fatty meats and fish. All plant foods contain carbohydrates but the main energy sources in our diet are sugar, flour and other cereals, and root vegetables such as potatoes. Between them these groups of foods provide nutrients that include vitamins and minerals, materials for growth and repair of body tissue and of course energy (often called calories).

Fibre does none of these things, so although it is present in some of the foods above, its significance has been ignored. It is the only component of our food that contains almost no calories. It is broken down by bacteria in the large bowel and provides some energy absorbed from there. And yet, if you think about it, there must be a role for a food that does what no other food can do – passing through the upper part of the gut, known as the small intestine, to enter the large intestine more or less in its original state. What, for instance, does its presence do to the contents of the large intestine? And even more significant at a time when our modern diet is very low in fibre, what is the effect of its absence in the bowel?

These questions are concerning many scientists today; therefore, in writing this book I have tried to set out in clear language the scientific evidence that has led to the change in attitude to the importance of fibre. I will describe how the implications of this new awareness can be practically applied, with simple, everyday dietary suggestions for protection against some of the most common Western diseases, including constipation, diverticular disease, hiatus hernia, appendicitis, varicose veins, piles, diabetes, coronary heart disease, bowel cancer and gall-stones.

In writing this book, I have deliberately not set out to make it a general work on diet, a task for which I would be quite unqualified. Instead I have concentrated on a component of food which has been almost totally neglected and have largely confined myself to aspects of nutrition in the study of which I have been personally involved. It is not a good policy to make supposedly authoritative statements without sufficient authority. Regrettably, dogmatic statements are often given by those who lack such authority.

Fortunately my medical background has given me particular opportunities to work in the field of dietary fibre. For twenty years I worked as a surgeon in Africa and during part of this time, and for the thirteen years since leaving Africa, I have been intensively studying on a world-wide basis the geographical distribution of many non-infectious diseases, including all those that will be discussed in this book. Initially my work was limited to cancer but during the last ten years I have been collecting material from all over the world on the geographical and cultural distribution of the characteristically Western diseases listed in chapter three.

Studies of the geographical distribution of these diseases have made it clear that many of them are rare and in some cases virtually unknown among traditionally-living peoples. There is also no evidence that these diseases were not relatively rare even in Western countries before the twentieth century.

There are, of course, many differences between the life-styles of traditionally living communities and our own; but there is strong evidence that dietary factors play a predominant role in causing many of these diseases. It is likely that there are multiple causes of each of them and other factors that may be protective against them. Although particular aspects of diet will be emphasized in this book, it is important to remember that it is the whole way of life rather than any single aspect that distinguishes traditional from advanced societies.

Some people have, from time to time, placed undue emphasis on one particular aspect of diet, but the general consensus of current scientific opinion would agree that the most harmful changes that have occurred in Western diets over the past century have been the replacement of carbohydrate foods, such as bread and other cereals, by fat (and animal fat in particular). Moreover carbohydrate foods which were previously eaten with their natural fibre content intact are now largely consumed depleted of fibre. In particular this applies to sugar which is totally devoid of fibre and to white flour from which most of the fibre is removed in modern milling processes. As a result there has been a much more marked fall in our consumption of cereal than of total fibre. Recent research has shown that fibre in cereals is much more effective than fibre in fruit and green vegetables in maintaining normal intestinal behaviour and content.

The importance of these findings is only beginning to be grasped by scientists throughout the world. A significantly increased intake of fibre-rich cereal foods could almost abolish the near-universal problem of constipation in Western communities and as a result might significantly reduce the prevalence of some of the diseases mentioned earlier. It must be emphasized when considering harmful changes in diet that Western communities were not necessarily better nourished a century ago, when malnutrition was rife among the poor.

Claims have so often been made, entirely without evidence, for the beneficial effects of certain foods, that it is not surprising that most doctors and their patients have viewed with caution the idea that dietary habits might profoundly influence disease patterns. The increasing recognition that many common diseases are related to a Western life-style, rather than to genetic factors, has prompted a search for carefully documented evidence of relationships between these diseases and dietary habits.

One of the first to recognize a relationship between refined carbohydrate foods and disease was Dr T.R. Allinson who, in an essay written nearly a century ago, related not only constipation but also piles (haemorrhoids) and varicose veins to an insufficiency of fibre in the diet. Sir Robert Macarrison, early in the 1900s, warned of the dangers of over-processing food. These observations did not receive serious attention until Surgeon Captain T.L. Cleave, a British naval physician with perceptive genius, persuasive argument and irrefutable logic not only linked together a number of diseases of unknown cause but presented compelling evidence that each of them might be only a different result of a common cause – the consumption of over-refined carbohydrate foods. Captain Cleave was also the first to demonstrate dramatically the beneficial effect of bran in combating constipation when he was chief medical officer and responsible for the health of the crew of the battle-ship *King George V* during the Second World War. It was he who first persuaded me of the profound influence of diet on patterns of disease.

In his book *The Saccharine Disease* he described his convictions that many of the characteristically Western diseases might be caused by over-consumption of refined carbohydrate foods, and of sugar in particular, hence the name saccharine meaning 'related to sugar'. This study involved writing letters longhand to thousands of doctors throughout the world, and thus amassing information on the geographical distribution of various diseases. The data collected compelled the conclusion that the refining of carbohydrate foods might be to a large extent responsible for many diseases characteristic of modern Western culture.

Meeting Captain Cleave was one of the most important occasions in my professional life. Background knowledge of disease patterns in the Third World enabled me to recognize instantly the undeniable truth and logic of his ideas. I also had unique opportunities through medical contacts in most of Africa and Asia to confirm or deny statements he had made, and as will be shown later in this book the mass of opinion endorsed his conclusions. Most of the medical profession at that time viewed Captain Cleave's ideas with scepticism, and consequently his evidence was rejected without proper consideration.

The recognition given by the medical profession to my earlier work describing a form of cancer to which my name was given (Burkitt's Lymphoma), provided me with opportunities that would not otherwise have been offered to communicate the concepts of Captain Cleave and others. Moreover, the numerous worldwide contacts I had established for collecting data on cancer distribution provided unique opportunities for testing the validity of these ideas. I was able for example to check the frequency of occurrence of specific diseases in different parts of the world by sending and receiving monthly questionnaires to over 140 rural hospitals mainly in Africa and India.

Pioneer work in scientific exploration serves as a foundation on which subsequent explorers build, and the contribution of the pioneer can be too easily overlooked and forgotten as the edifice grows. Maps made by early navigators invariably have been enormously modified by subsequent cartographers, but this detracts nothing from the contribution of the original discoverer. So it has been with medical discovery.

The original ideas put forward by Cleave and others will stand as landmarks in medical history but details have been, and will continue to be, altered in the light of ever-emerging new facts. Many of the conclusions drawn from evidence currently available and presented in this book are still hypotheses that have not yet reached the status of confirmed fact. These hypotheses may well be changed following further research and future findings.

It is not uncommon for people who write on health and other subjects to begin with an emotionally derived conviction and then selectively to look for evidence which will support their preconceived opinions. I have a card on my desk with the all-too-common attitude printed on it, 'My mind is made up, don't confuse me with facts.' Even with scientists, commendable enthusiasm can fall into this trap, and I am far from immune, although acutely aware of the difference between provisional hypothesis and proven fact.

In order to emphasize the weight of evidence showing the dominant role of dietary factors as a cause of certain diseases the next two chapters will deal with the principles of the interpretation of this evidence. The techniques of epidemiology, by which is meant the geographical and socio-economic distribution of a disease, and the relationships between a disease and particular factors in the environment will be outlined.

Some readers may prefer to move straight on to the main argument of this book — the relationship between a deficiency of fibre in diet and some of our commonest diseases. If you are less interested in finding out how scientists examine these subjects, than in the conclusions they reach, skip the next two chapters and go straight to chapter three.

1 WHAT CAUSES DISEASE?

Where we are and what we are

The vast majority of illnesses are the result of where we are, and the environmental circumstances that surround us, rather than of any inherent defect in our make-up. We are constantly being influenced by a multitude of seen and unseen things – the sun's rays, the food and drink that enter our body and the air we breath. In addition we are exposed to hostile attack by other creatures and also by our fellow men.

On the other hand we have, built into our systems, elaborate and beautifully designed mechanisms to counter the attack of a huge variety of bacteria and parasites that may invade our bodies. We are partially protected by the pigment in our skin from the effects of excessive sun radiation and by the reflex mechanisms that take instantaneous and automatic action at the approach of danger. An example is the way we immediately close our eyelids when anything touches our eyes.

People of different ethnic groups usually suffer from the same diseases when living in the same environment, whereas those from the same groups, if living in different environments, suffer from different diseases, depending on the harmful factors to which they are exposed in those environments.

The balance of health

Too often disease is viewed merely as the result of harmful influences, while factors that protect from disease are overlooked. Both sickness and health are dependant on a balance between beneficial and harmful

14

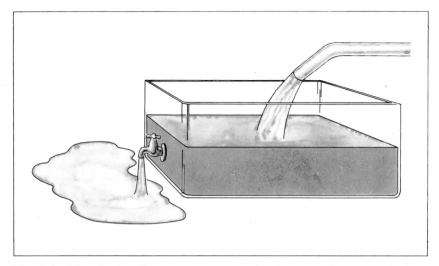

The risk of developing disease, represented by the level of the water in the tank, depends on the relative amounts entering and leaving, depicting causative and protective factors.

influences, between the effectiveness of the things that attack us and the ability of our bodies to defend themselves. The situation can be compared to a conflict between two opposing armies. If one of the armies is depleted, it will have an effect on the outcome of the battle, as will augmenting the opposing forces. Although many of our general protective mechanisms against disease are inbuilt before birth, we can develop particular defences against specific diseases as a result of successfully combating attacks by the organisms which produce these diseases.

The balance between attacking and defending forces in our bodies can be compared to a water tank with one pipe supplying water to it and another draining water from it (above). The level of the water in the tank depends on the relative amount flowing from each tap. The water entering can be taken to represent the cause of a disease, the outflow the protective mechanisms, and the level of water the risk of developing disease. The higher the level – the greater the risk. Increasing the inflow or reducing the outflow will have the same effect and vice versa.

Bodies like the Food and Drugs Administration in the United States are right to be careful to ensure that potentially harmful substances are not added to food, but how much thought is given to the removal of potentially protective components of food?

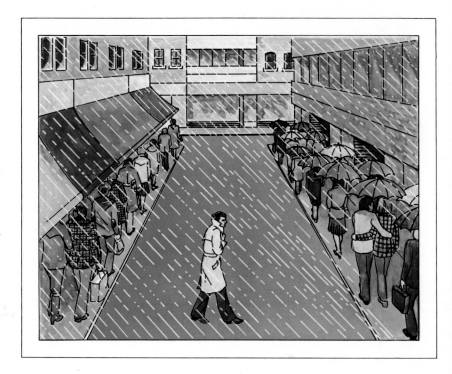

All animals, including man, tend to adapt to any hostile elements in the environment in which they live, so that in time they develop mechanisms which protect them against these dangers. For example, animals develop body colours which blend with their environment and thus provide protection through camouflage. In a similar way polar animals develop furry coats that effectively insulate them against the cold.

Men or animals who are not normally exposed to certain hostile environments do not require protection against them. They are like the men on the left of the illustration (above) who are under shelter, so do not require umbrellas to protect them from the rain. Rain is falling around those on the right of the illustration but these people remain dry, that is disease free, because they have acquired protection in the form of umbrellas. If a man without an umbrella walks from shelter into the rain he gets wet. The rain in the illustration represents an environment capable of causing a disease to develop. The people under shelter are not exposed to the environment so remain dry, that is disease free. Those who are in the harmful environment of the rain and have acquired the protective immunity of the umbrellas also remain dry, that is free of disease. Those who go into the harmful environment without this protection get wet; that is they will develop the disease.

Some people, because of their genetically inherited make-up, are more susceptible to certain disease-producing influences than are others. If once again we compare the environment in which we find ourselves to rain, and our protection against disease to umbrellas, our chances of keeping dry will depend not only on the possession of an umbrella but also on its size, that is, the extent of the protection that we have against the hostile environment. An understanding of this principle of adaptation to environment is very relevant to the main argument of this book which deals with the diseases characteristic of modern Western man.

We have already seen that most disease is caused by environment, and even defects present at birth can be the result of some harmful factor during the baby's development in the womb. A good example of this is the tragedy of the deformities caused to the unborn child by the mother taking the drug thalidomide. There are also a few diseases which are transmitted genetically from parent to child.

Changing patterns of disease

Environmental causes of disease are very varied. The major cause is infection from bacteria and parasites of different kinds. Causes of the different infective diseases are now largely known, and consequently energetic measures have been highly successful in controlling most of them. As a result in Western countries the pattern of disease has dramatically changed over the past century. A hundred years ago by far the commonest causes of illness and death were infective diseases such as pneumonia, gastro-enteritis, diptheria, tuberculosis and meningitis. Deaths from these causes are relatively rare today. These and other infective diseases are, however, still the major cause of sickness and death in the Third World.

The major health hazards, providing the commonest causes of death in Western countries today, are the non-infective diseases whose causes are still, or have until recently been, unknown. These include cancer, arterial disease and other so-called 'degenerative' diseases. They are however all rare in Third World countries, even among the elderly.

17

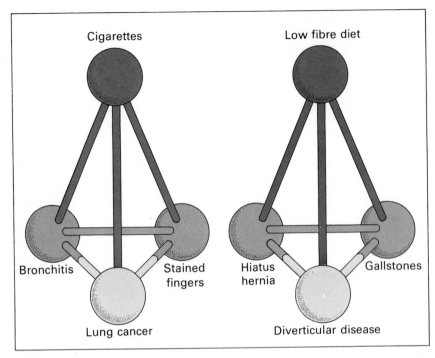

The effects of a common cause are associated.

Because of this new realization the name 'degenerative' hardly seems appropriate.

Weighing up the causes

It is important to recognize that many different factors may contribute to the cause of any one disease. Coronary heart disease is probably a good example. Male sex, smoking and consumption of large quantities of fats are regarded as high risk factors, whereas exercise and fibre-rich foods have been claimed to be protective. It is possible to reduce the risk of a disease by getting rid of a major cause. For example giving up smoking will drastically reduce lung cancer but not totally eliminate it as there are other causes. All the effects of a common cause are associated with each other. Consequently, associations found between diseases suggest they share a common cause (see diagram above).

The situation can also be compared to the balance of weighing scales. On one side you have the causative factors of disease, represented by one pan of the scales. On the other, there are the various protective factors. When the causative ones outweigh the protective factors forcing the first pan down – disease occurs.

Not only can several different factors contribute to the cause of a single disease, but a single factor may contribute to the cause of a number of apparently different diseases, which in certain circumstances may be viewed as different aspects of a single disease – as they share a common cause. For example, typhoid fever, which used to be common in Western countries and is still common in tropical regions, can show itself in many different forms, some appearing long after the acute phase of the disease is over. It gives rise not only to fever, a skin rash, abdominal pain and changes in the blood in its early stages, but subsequent effects include changes within the bones, gall-bladder disease and arthritis. Each of these might well have been considered to be a different disease before the underlying cause of each – the bacteria responsible for causing typhoid fever – was identified. Once the basic cause had been identified, it became possible to protect against it.

Later in this book I will show how relevant these basic principles and simple illustrations are to discovering the causes of, and the means of prevention from, some of our commonest diseases.

2 HOW ENVIRONMENT PLAYS A PART

What contributes to health?

Life expectancy at birth in Western countries is much greater today than it was a century or more ago. This is much more the result of clean water supplies, satisfactory sewage disposal, adequate nutrition, ample clothing and shelter than of therapeutic medicine. Although infant mortality has fallen enormously during this century (right), life expectancy in middle age has scarcely increased at all during this period. This is largely because relatively new diseases, including those to be discussed in this book, have taken the place of infective diseases as a major cause of death.

In 1950 less than one medical prescription was issued per person per year in Australia; the figure today has risen to over ten. Yet during this time there has been no appreciable change in life expectancy after middle age in spite of the enormously increased availability of potent drugs to combat infection.

It is true that new drugs such as certain antibiotics played a significant role in treating tuberculosis – once a major scourge in Western countries, but improved food, housing and sanitation led to a dramatic fall in mortality before modern drugs became available.

In Western countries today diseases produced by bacterial infections are no longer a major cause of death as they were a century and more ago. Their place as major causes of death and disability has been taken by the so-called 'degenerative' diseases. Now that these diseases have been shown not to be common in old age in less developed communities the word degenerative is no longer strictly applicable. Improvement in

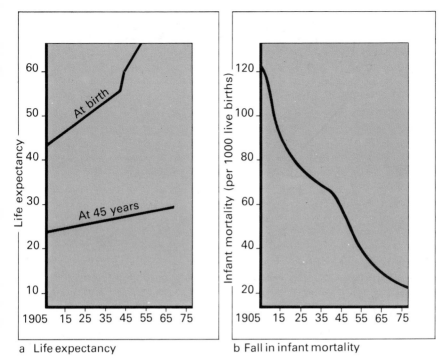

a Life expectancy   b Fall in infant mortality

a   The higher life expectancy at birth due to the fall in infant mortality
     from 1905 to 1975 showing the minimal increase in life expectancy at
     45 years old.
b   The fall in infant mortality from 1905 to 1975 in England and Wales.

hygiene, cleaner water and milk supplies and adequate nutrition,
assisted by more effective drugs, played a major role in combating
infectious disease. Fortunately as will be shown in this chapter, a very
useful method of looking at modern disease has been evolved which
points the way to a better understanding of the underlying causes of
non-infective diseases.

Geographical distribution –
a clue to the cause of disease

Most diseases are caused by harmful factors in the environment, so it
follows that a high incidence of a disease in a certain area or among a
particular group of people may point to some local causative factor. If
people of different races in a particular environment get a certain
disease, but in a different environment are all free from this disease, it

21

can be concluded that the cause of the disease lies in the environment and not in the genetic make-up of the different people.

The study of the geographical or socio-economic distribution of disease is called epidemiology. One of the most fruitful ways of discovering the cause of a disease is by studying its pattern of distribution and then considering possible disease-causing factors with the same distribution. In this way many clues will emerge. If two or more diseases are caused by the same factor they will have the same geographical or socio-economic distribution. Conversely if two diseases have the same distribution it suggests that they are probably the result, at least in part, of the same cause. One classic example of this approach is John Snow's discovery of the cause of cholera. In a cholera epidemic Snow plotted on a street map of London the distribution of cholera cases and then searched for some factor that was common to them all and which might link them together. He found that they all drew their water from the same pump in Broad Street. The water from this pump was drawn from the River Thames below the entry of sewage disposal and was thus contaminated with human excreta. Not till many years later was the organism responsible for cholera identified.

Another example of discovering the cause of a disease by relating its distribution to environmental factors comes from the study of cancer. Sir Percival Pott, over a century ago, recognized that many of the elderly men consulting him with skin cancer had been employed as chimney sweeps as young boys, at a time when children were sent up chimneys to remove the soot. He related the cancer to skin contact with soot-impregnated clothes long before it became known that soot contains substances that can be powerful carcinogens (cancer-forming substances).

It is important to remember that both Snow and Pott recognized causative associations between diseases and particular factors in the environment long before the ways in which they produced disease became understood. They were able to advise means of prevention without waiting until science provided proof that the suspected factors were in fact causes of the associated diseases.

Relationships between diseases

Different diseases may share the same causes and they will consequently

22

tend to occur in the same individuals. The typhoid fever example, mentioned in chapter one, illustrates this. The many different clinical manifestations of the disease associated in the same patients suggested they might share a common cause.

When one disease follows another it is sometimes wrongly assumed that the second is caused by, and is a complication of, the first. An alternative explanation may well be that both diseases are due to a common cause, and that the second to appear requires more time to develop than does the first. It may be that factor X causes disease A, then disease A causes disease B.

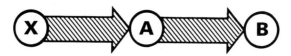

Alternatively both A and B may be independent results of the common cause of X but that A appears before B.

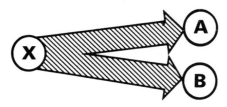

Naturally, if you are trying to find factor X you have to look for reasonable links between the environment and diseases represented by A and B. In some countries the increase in lung cancer might be related to the number of television sets, but this does not necessarily imply that television viewing causes lung cancer. To return to our analogy of the pipe filling the tank. A tank may have a pipe leading into it from which no water is flowing; therefore this pipe could not influence the water level of the tank. Or the tank can have a pipe leading into it from which water is flowing which will influence the water level. The former is a non-causative and the latter a causative relationship.

Age is a factor that determines susceptibility to disease. This is partly because the longer you live the more exposed you are to detrimental factors in the environment and partly because defence mechanisms against disease become weaker in old age.

It is often incorrectly assumed that because life expectancy at birth in poorer countries may be only forty years this implies that there are few old people. It is, however, mainly the high infant mortality that lowers the average expectancy at birth — rather than death in middle life. Although there are significantly fewer old people in Third-World countries than in Western communities there are plenty of them, and the rarity of many of the diseases discussed in this book cannot therefore be explained by a lack of elderly people in the population.

The distribution in the population of people of different ages in India and the United States shows that the lower life expectancy at birth is influnced much more by the high infant mortality than by people failing to reach old age. Although there are fewer old people than in Western countries, the proportion of people over the age of fifty years is only about two and a half times greater in the United States despite the far greater proportion surviving childhood. If a disease characteristic of old age is, say, three times as common in Western countries as in Third-World communities, the age discrepancy might account for it but certainly not when the discrepancy is between ten and over one hundred times as it is in the case of the diseases discussed in this book.

With this in mind, we will, in the next chapter, look at the distribution of some of the typically Western diseases round the world, comparing their occurrence in developed and in underdeveloped countries.

3 CAN SOME OF OUR COMMONEST AILMENTS BE PREVENTED?

World-wide comparisons

Once you begin to compare the occurrence of some of our most common diseases with their incidence in other parts of the world you start to find dramatic differences. These differences will be described here but possible reasons for this wide variation will be considered in chapters four and five.

Coronary heart disease

This is the commonest cause of death in Western countries, killing about one man in four. It is also an increasingly important cause of death among elderly women. It was a rare disease even in Western countries until after the First World War. Coronary heart disease is also almost unknown among rural Africans and is uncommon in most rural communities in Asia. In African cities only occasional cases are found and these are always among the most Westernized part of the community. It was much less common among black than white Americans forty and more years ago, yet black and white Americans living in similar circumstances are comparably affected by this disease today.

Gallstones

Removal of the gall-bladder is currently one of the most frequently performed abdominal operations in Western countries and gallstones have become commoner during this century. They are exceedingly rare in Africa, where many hospitals may not see even one patient with gallstones in ten years.

The Pima Indians in the south-west of the United States have been found to have a higher frequency of gallstones than any other group. Over 70 per cent of Pima Indian women between twenty-five and forty have gallstones. They are present in over 20 per cent of women over the age of thirty in most Western countries.

Diverticular disease of the colon
This is the commonest disorder of the large intestine. It is present, though usually without symptoms, in one in ten people over the age of forty, and in one in three over the age of sixty. Even in Western countries it was rarely reported before the late 1920s. Of all the modern diseases this is the rarest in Third-World communities. It is almost unknown in Africa and in Asia. The few cases observed in Asian countries have for the most part been in the top socio-economic levels of the community. Only occasional cases are observed even in large university clinics in India.

Appendicitis
This is the most frequent cause for emergency abdominal surgery. About one person in eight has had his or her appendix removed by middle age. As with the diseases listed above, the frequency of appendicitis greatly increased in Western countries during the early years of the present century, before reaching a fairly stationary level. It became less common in European countries during the Second World War when there was food rationing. It was almost unknown to doctors in many of the prisoner-of-war camps.

In Africa and Asia appendicitis is a disease of urban populations and of upper socio-economic groups rather than of peasant rural communities. We taught our Ugandan doctors that they should be wary about diagnosing appendicitis in an African unless he could speak English. This was an index of his contact with Western culture!

In the past when food in British prisons was coarser than that eaten outside, appendicitis was less common among prisoners than in the rest of the population.

Presumably it was not found among American slaves when they were brought from rural Africa, but it had become fairly common among black Americans forty or fifty years ago. Appendicitis is as common now among black as white Americans.

Hiatus hernia

This is an upward protrusion of the top of the stomach through the hole in the diaphragm that contains the oesophagus or gullet and into the thoracic cavity (see page 58). It can be demonstrated by taking an X-ray after the person has eaten a meal containing barium which is radio-opaque in about one in five adults. In the majority of hiatus hernia cases there are no symptoms. In a number, however, it is associated with heartburn, due to the entry of gastric acid up into the gullet. Hiatus hernia is very rare among traditionally living people. A radiological study in West Africa revealed only four cases in over a thousand who were carefully examined for the presence of this defect. Similar figures have been reported from other parts of Africa. It is a little commoner in Asian communities but still rare compared with Western countries.

Varicose veins

A community-wide study in Michigan in the United States showed that 44 per cent of women between the ages of thirty and fifty had varicose veins compared to 24 per cent of men of the same group. The same study found 64 per cent of women over fifty had them compared to 42 per cent of men. Varicose veins are much less common in developing countries and are particularly rare among people who have had minimal contact with Western culture. Varicose veins have been estimated to be present in under 5 per cent of rural Africans and Indians. Their prevalence in different groups of Pacific Islands is directly related to contact with Western culture. Varicose veins are even more common among New Zealand Maori women than white women, and equally common among black and white Americans today.

In Asia varicose veins are more common among trishaw riders who ride a tricycle which carries passengers seated behind than they are among barbers who stand at their work. The former are subject to considerable abdominal straining as they pedal. These examples show that environmental factors are more important than genetic ones in causing this disorder.

Piles (haemorrhoids)

This is one of the most common ailments to which Western man is prone. Piles have been reported to be present in one out of every two Americans over the age of fifty. They are much less common in

Third-World countries and are relatively rare among tribal communities

Large bowel cancer
This is the most common cause of cancer death in North America and in Britain today with the exception of lung cancer due to cigarette smoking. There is no other type of cancer so closely related to economic development and our way of life. It is far more common in Western communities than it is in populations in the Third World.

In North America there are two religious groups who suffer about a third less bowel cancer than other Americans. These are the Seventh Day Adventists who are predominantly vegetarian, and Mormons who are not. These two groups also have a comparably lower risk of developing coronary heart disease and, being non-smokers, are almost completely free from lung cancer.

Although they live in a comparable culture, rural Finns have only about a quarter of the incidence of bowel cancer as Copenhagen Danes or New Yorkers.

Diabetes
This is the most common disorder of the endocrine glands. It is present, though not necessarily detected, in about 5 per cent of English adults under fifty and about 15 per cent over fifty. It has not yet been reported among any pure-blooded hunter-food gatherers, such as African bushmen, Laplanders and so on. One of the most striking examples of the way in which this disease is related to a modern Western life-style is provided by the little island of Nauru in the Pacific.

A few years ago it was discovered that the whole island was covered with phosphates, obviously of great economic value. As a result its people are now among the wealthiest in the world. They import Western-type food, lead a leisurely life, and already over 30 per cent of the population over the age of fifteen suffer from diabetes, whereas once the incidence of the disease was as low as it is in other Pacific islands. They are increasingly suffering from appendicitis, another disease to emerge relatively early after impact with Western culture. Coronary heart disease and gallstones will almost certainly emerge in time. Diseases like hiatus hernia and diverticular disease will not be expected until after at least a generation.

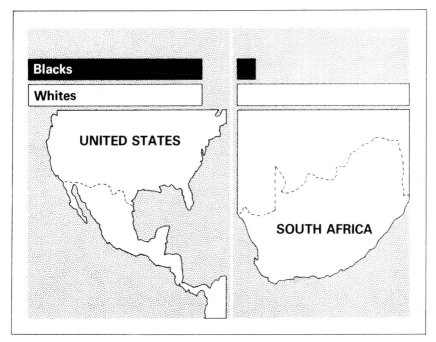

The blocks represent the occurrence of the diseases described in the previous diagram. They occur just as frequently among white Americans as among black Americans and white South Africans. Black South Africans are rarely affected.

Another striking example of the effect of environment on diabetes is provided by the Indians in South Africa whose forebears emigrated from south India. They now get about ten times as much diabetes as Indians who live in India.

Obesity

At least 40 per cent of middle-aged adults in North America and Western Europe are overweight. This is rarely a problem among tribal communities where weight increases little after early adult life. Indeed in primitive communities body weight falls during middle age although it rises in all Western communities.

All the diseases listed in this chapter are rare among black South Africans but affect white South Africans to approximately the same extent as Americans. Yet in the United States they affect blacks and

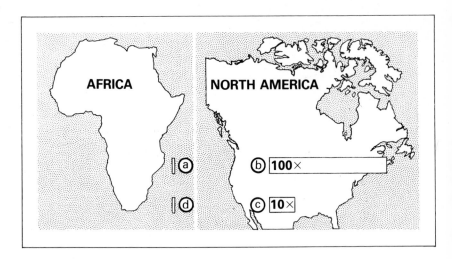

Blocks **a** and **b** represent the occurrence of coronary heart disease, diverticular disease, gallstones, appendicitis and hiatus hernia in areas like North America **a** and rural Africa **b**.
They occur 100 times more frequently in **a** than **b**.
Varicose veins, piles, large bowel cancer, diabetes and obesity, represented by blocks **c** and **d** occur ten times more frequently in areas like North America than rural Africa.

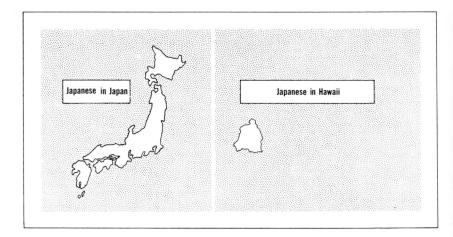

These diseases were relatively rare in Japan until after the Second World War. They are still much less common there than in the US, but are increasing in Japanese cities.
Within a generation of Japanese emigrating to Hawaii the occurrence of these diseases has become comparable to that among other Americans.

30

whites more or less equally (left, above). They were presumably as rare or rarer among American slaves as they are today in the parts of Africa from which the slaves came. Forty or more years ago the diseases, for which information was available, were much less common among black than white Americans, but both groups are now equally affected today.

These diseases were uncommon in Japan until after the Second World War, but are now increasing rapidly. Japanese who emigrated to Hawaii and California and adopted an American way of life have, within a generation, become almost equally prone to develop these diseases as other Americans (left, below).

From the above information we are forced to draw the inescapable conclusion that these common diseases are primarily the result of a man-made environment rather than genetic in origin. If we could only identify and eradicate or minimize their causes these diseases would be largely preventable.

Not only do they have similar geographical and socio-economic distributions, but many of them tend to occur together in individual patients. These observations suggest that the diseases described all share some common cause although this need not be the only one. Alternatively some factor in the environment may provide protection against each of these diseases.

In the following chapters we will consider which factors in these contrasting environments are most likely to be responsible for causing or protecting against these diseases. The first step in the prevention of any disease is, of course, identification of its cause, and a study of these possible factors will give us some clues.

4 LOOK TO YOUR DIET

Changing eating patterns

In the last chapter it was shown that a formidable list of diseases is common in Western countries but rarely found in less developed parts of the world. Even in Western countries most of them have only become widespread during the last sixty or so years. Therefore the main causes must lie in some aspects of our modern way of life.

I will show in later chapters that most of the diseases mentioned are related either directly or indirectly to the behaviour of the gut (known as the intestinal tract) as food passes along it. In view of the staggering disparity in the frequency of these diseases in Western and in Third-World countries, is seems logical as a next step to compare the usual dietary habits in the places where they are rarely found with those of communities most affected.

When food is prepared in a simple way such as grinding grain by hand between two stones , or pounding it in a wooden tub, and the product is then eaten with little extracted or removed from it, all the diseases mentioned are relatively rare. The earliest changes in diet that take place in Third-World countries as they begin to develop economically are usually the introduction of sugar, sweetened drinks and white bread in place of the minimally-processed carbohydrate foods that previously provided the staple diet. The eating pattern changes towards

RIGHT: Stone-grinding removes none of the fibre, minerals or vitamins extracted in the manufacture of white flour. Mass production of wholemeal flour would not require a reversion to stone mills but could be made using suitably adjusted modern machinery.

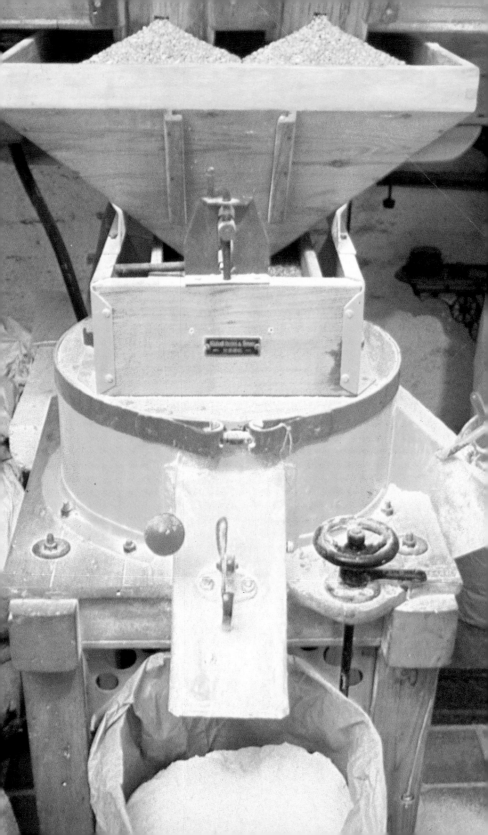

the style of a typical Western diet where fat plays a prominant role, sugar intake increases (pages 35 and 36) and consumption of little-processed starchy foods such as whole grains and potatoes is considerably reduced.

This means there are fundamental changes in the proportions of energy (or calories) derived from the three main food components: protein, carbohydrate and fat (see page 35). The differences between the food consumed in Western communities today and that eaten by rural populations in the Third World are similar to the differences between Western diets today compared to the food our ancestors ate a century or more ago.

The proportion of energy derived from protein is fairly constant, usually varying somewhere between 10 and 15 per cent. Its nature, however, changes from being mainly derived from vegetable foods in developing countries to being largely of animal origin in more affluent societies. Fat intake rises with economic development so that Western communities eat three or four times as much fat as do people in poorer countries. In addition its nature changes, as in the case of protein, with animal fat largely replacing vegetable fat.

Along with the rise in fat consumption goes a change both in overall carbohydrate intake and also in the kind of carbohydrates eaten. In rural communities in the Third World carbohydrate provides between 70 and 80 per cent of energy (calories), and is consumed with its full comple-ment of fibre, the undigestible portion consisting largely of plant cell walls. In Western countries the fibre content has been largely extracted in the manufacture of sugar and highly refined white flour. The latter has replaced brown and wholemeal flour which is rich in fibre. Modern milling methods strip away the outer layers of the grain. Refined sugar, which is almost entirely composed of energy (calories), and white flour now provide much of our reduced carbohydrate consumption. The average annual sugar intake in Western countries of about 120 lb (58 kg) is about ten times that in poorer countries. Consumption of potatoes has also fallen in Western countries.

The significance of fibre

The food component that changes most with adoption of Western dietary habits is the indigestible fibre. Two and a half times more fibre, approximately $1\frac{1}{2}$ to 2 oz (40 to 60 g) daily is consumed in Third-World

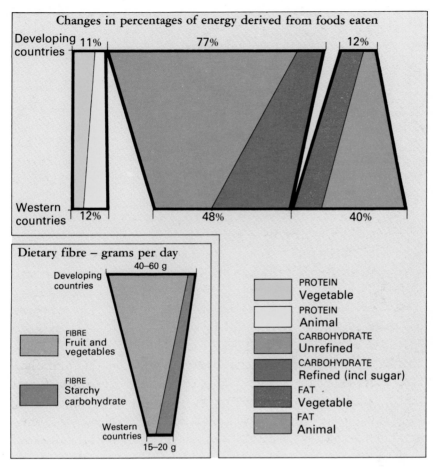

Changes in percentages of energy derived from foods eaten

Developing countries: 11% | 77% | 12%

Western countries: 12% | 48% | 40%

Dietary fibre – grams per day

Developing countries: 40–60 g

Western countries: 15–20 g

FIBRE Fruit and vegetables

FIBRE Starchy carbohydrate

PROTEIN Vegetable

PROTEIN Animal

CARBOHYDRATE Unrefined

CARBOHYDRATE Refined (incl sugar)

FAT Vegetable

FAT Animal

ABOVE: The relative proportion of energy (calories) provided by protein, carbohydrate and fat in Third World compared to Western countries.

BELOW: Changes in fibre intake both overall and in source.

countries than in Western communities, in which considerably less than 1 oz (15 to 25 g) is eaten daily. The difference may not sound enormous but for the way the body works is has great significance, in view of the fact that relatively minor changes operating over many years can produce major effects. There is a difference in the nature of the foods from which we derive our fibre. In Western countries it is derived mainly from fruit and leaf vegetables whereas in Third-World countries it is mostly provided by cereal foods and root vegetables.

These increases and decreases in food components can be illustrated in another way. Whereas total protein intake in affluent communities is

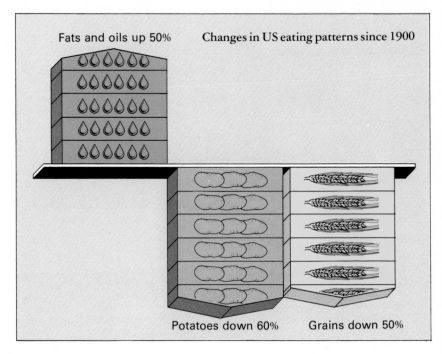

Fats and oils up 50%   Changes in US eating patterns since 1900

Potatoes down 60%   Grains down 50%

Sugar consumption has increased to an even greater extent.

only moderately more than in poor countries the proportion derived from animal sources is seven times greater. While fat intake in the Western diet is about three times greater than that of poor countries the proportion derived from animal sources is eight times greater. The difference in sugar intake can be as great as ten-fold.

In contrast to these dramatic *increases* in food intake there has been a similarly dramatic *reduction* in fibre intake in affluent countries to only about one third (30 to 40 per cent) that of poorer countries in Africa and Asia. Fibre intake is reduced as fat and sugar consumption increases (see page 87). As consumption of fats, oils and sugar has increased the consumption of grains and potatoes has decreased (above).

The fibre reduction is greater than the carbohydrate reduction. When carbohydrate foods provide a high proportion of the total energy (calories) consumed in the daily diet they are lightly processed foods which are relatively rich in fibre. When they provide a smaller proportion of energy more of them are highly processed cereal foods, such as white flour or white rice, with less fibre.

36

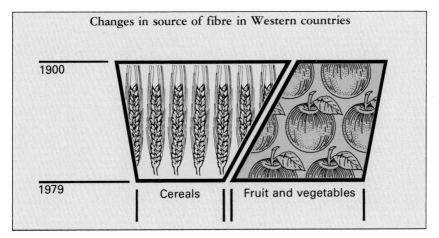

The proportion of fibre provided by cereals has been reduced, while that from fruit and vegetables has increased.

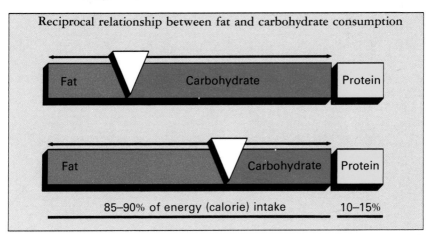

As pointed out in the last chapter, fibre from fruits and vegetables has, over the past century, increased in Western countries whereas fibre from cereals has decreased (see above). Although the total consumption of fibre has not altered greatly in Western countries, recent research has emphasized that cereal fibre present in wholemeal bread, coarse oatmeal, rye crispbread, brown rice and bran is more likely to be effective in preventing certain diseases than an equal amount of fibre derived from fruit and vegetables. This will be discussed in more detail in chapter twelve.

As an example of the effect of this difference, studies of the diet of South African Bantu have shown that their fibre intake is over four times that of Western communities. This would almost certainly be true of all communities in sub-Saharan Africa among whom virtually all the Western diseases are invariably rare.

We have already seen that fat and carbohydrate intake are reciprocally related and this is an exceedingly important fact. Together they provide between 85 and 90 per cent of energy in most communities, so that a high fat diet is inevitably a low carbohydrate diet and vice versa (see previous page). Since reduction in carbohydrate is accompanied by a much greater reduction in fibre, fibre intake and fat intake are inevitably inversely related. As intake of fat goes up, that of carbohydrate and fibre goes down.

In Western countries today sugar, which is pure energy, accounts for about 50 per cent of our energy derived from carbohydrate foods. Sugar has partially replaced the fibre-rich cereals; tubers, including potatoes and parsnips; legumes, including peas and beans, which could be easily stored and were eaten in larger quantities previously. Now most of our reduced fibre-intake comes from fruit and vegetables.

Consequent on the reciprocal relationship between fat and fibre intake evidence that points to an increase in fat consumption as a cause of any disease must inevitably point equally strongly to a decrease in fibre. Neither of these opposite sides of the coin should be viewed in isolation. The more bulky fibre-rich foods you eat the less fat you will be consuming, and vice versa. At its simplest, if you eat more fibre-rich foods they are bulkier and fill the stomach up while providing less energy than foods that are rich in calories like sugar and fat. How this happens will be shown in a later chapter when we come to look at how obesity occurs (chapter eleven).

5 FIBRE -
THE FORGOTTEN FACTOR

We have now looked at the main energy-providing components of our diet — protein, fat and carbohydrate. There are of course other requirements such as vitamins and small quantities of elements such as zinc, iron and calcium.

Nutritionists have given much thought to these three major energy-containing, calorie-rich components of food. The largely non-nutritious portion, the fibre, has been misunderstood, neglected and rejected for too long. Because it provides virtually no energy, fibre has been viewed as being of no value in food and its removal was believed to improve the quality of plant foods and of cereals in particular. It has in fact been regarded as a contaminant and consequently discarded to be used as animal feed. Although some individuals have in the past recognized this approach as being wrong, only in recent years has the fallacy of this assumption been scientifically demonstrated and consequently widely recognized among food scientists.

What is fibre and why is it important?

Fibre is the skeleton of the plant, without which no flower or tree would be able to stand upright. The walls of every cell are composed of fibre. The contents of a cell are the nutrients, the cell wall is their carton or container. Nutritionists have examined in detail the content but ignored the carton (page 40, above).

The fibre is more abundant on the outside of seeds, fruits, legumes

39

Plant cell

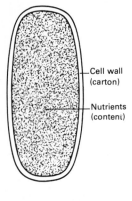

Cell wall (carton)

Nutrients (content)

Grain of wheat

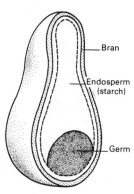

Bran

Endosperm (starch)

Germ

(peas and beans) and other foods than on the inside, and with the removal of the outside layers in milling and peeling much of the all-important fibre is discarded. Fibre is also removed when the content of cells is extracted and the cell wall removed as in the extraction of sugar from cane or beet; also when vegetable oils and fats are extracted from oil seeds, cereals and nuts.

Fibre is not a single substance, but is basically a mixture of three groups of substances. One is cellulose (a polysaccharide), another is lignin, which provides the woody part of plants. It is the only part of fibre that is not carbohydrate. There is a separate group of polysaccharides composed mainly of sugars, called pentoses, but including pectin (the setting agent in jams) and also gums, which are present in certain beans. The entire mix has been likened to ferro-concrete used for building construction, with cellulose representing the long straight iron bars; pentoses the branched-rods; the more soluble pectins and gums corresponding to the cement; and the lignin forming the tough outer covering.

It is interesting to note that at one time fibre was almost entirely equated with cellulose whereas it is now recognized that this is one of its less important constituents. The use of the term 'crude fibre' denoted only that part of plant food which was not broken down by boiling successively in weak acid and weak alkali. This, in fact, measured only part of the cellulose and part of the lignin (which gives woods its hardness), and none of those components that are now known to be so important in protecting against disease. Until recently, when fibre values were given in analyses of food contents, it was the crude-fibre element only that was included.

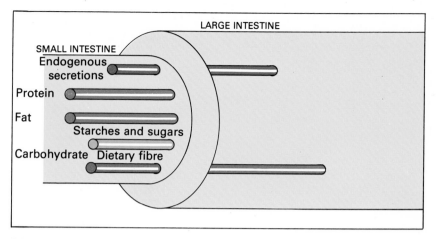

Dietary fibre reaches the large intestine intact

Fibre affects the function of the whole of the alimentary tract but it exerts its greatest influence in the large intestine, also known as the large bowel (which includes the colon and rectum). The simplest definition of fibre – now often called 'dietary fibre' by scientists – is the part of plant food that passes through the small intestine completely undigested and reaches the large intestine intact (above). Unlike fibre, nearly all of the starches, sugars, fats and protein eaten are digested and absorbed from the intestinal contents during their passage through the small intestine.

What happens to fibre in the body?

The accompanying diagram (on page 42) shows the passage of food from its entry into the mouth through to the elimination of residue in the stools. The food is broken up and mixed with saliva in the mouth. From there it passes through the oesophagus (gullet) to reach the stomach. Here it is mixed with digestive juices before being squeezed by the muscles in the wall of the stomach into the small intestine. Here it is mixed with other digestive juices which break it down into simpler chemical substances that can be absorbed into the veins carrying the nutrients and energy (calories) to the liver. In the liver it is prepared for various uses in the body.

Some of the food which is not absorbed in the small intestine is

The digestive system

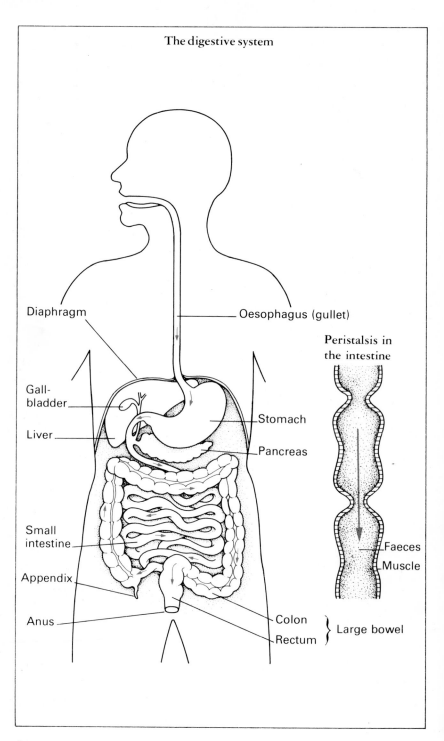

Diaphragm

Oesophagus (gullet)

Gall-bladder

Liver

Stomach

Pancreas

Peristalsis in the intestine

Small intestine

Appendix

Anus

Faeces

Muscle

Colon

Rectum

Large bowel

fermented by bacteria in the large intestine; products of this process are absorbed into the body. The rhythmic contractions of the gut or intestines, known as peristalsis, propel the bowel content through the intestine, rather like the gyrating movement of an earthworm. The bowel content is concentrated during its passage through the large bowel from being initially fluid into a solid or semi-solid state, excreted as stools. As defined above only fibre remains undigested in the small intestine and passes on to the large intestine relatively intact.

Fibre in food provides non-calorie-containing bulk, so you can increase the amount of fibre in your daily diet without increasing consumption of energy-rich foods. Fibre-rich foods require more chewing than do those depleted of their fibre. As a result they put a brake on the intake of energy and this will be discussed in chapter eleven when we look at obesity. Low-fibre foods leave the stomach more quickly to enter the intestine.

Fibre, by making the intestinal content more viscous, slows down the rate at which starch and sugar are absorbed and enter the bloodstream largely in the form of glucose. This in turn controls the demands put on the pancreas, the organ which produces the insulin needed for the digestion of glucose. The significance of this will be discussed in more detail when considering the cause of diabetes.

In the small and the large intestine, fibre interacts with cholesterol and bile salts, each of which are involved in causing both gallstones and coronary heart disease, again to be discussed in later chapters

Most of the large intestine consists of the colon. The last six inches or so is the rectum. When the undigested fibre arrives at this part of the gut, it has many important functions. Here the fibre interacts with various poisonous substances in the faeces (the name given to the content of the bowel), and prevents their absorption into the circulation of the body. In this way poisonous substances are eliminated from the body instead of being absorbed. If carcinogens (the substances which produce cancer), are diluted in a large volume of stool and also if they are discarded out of the bowel fairly quickly rather than hanging around, they will be less dangerous.

This has been demonstrated in experiments. If animals are fed a diet containing various poisons but rich in fibre, the poisons do little harm in certain doses. If the animals are fed the same poisons in the same doses but with a diet depleted of fibre, they sicken and die.

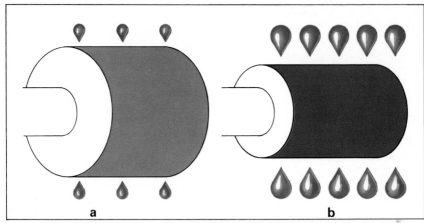

a Fibre leads to more water being retained in the intestine keeping the faeces soft and bulky.

b Low-fibre diets allow over-absorption of water from the intestinal content leading to a small volume of hard stools.

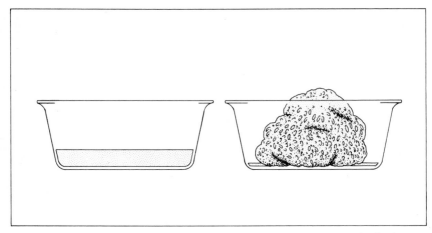

Fibre acts like a sponge retaining water and other constituents in the large bowel.

Probably the most important function of fibre in the colon is its ability to hold water in the form of a gel, like the way water is retained in seaweed or a bath sponge. This prevents the over-absorption of water from the intestinal content into the circulation (see illustration, above). Fibre in fact acts as an absorber, mopping up water and other constituents of the faeces (see lower illustration).

The liquid bowel content that enters the large intestine from the small intestine is thickened and made denser in the colon by the removal of water. When fibre is deficient too much water is removed so that the stools become small and firm. This water-holding capacity of fibre ensures that the bowel content remains large in volume and soft in consistency. Lack of fibre, and of cereal fibre in particular, is much the most important single cause of constipation, and the restoration of fibre to the diet is without doubt the most important means of combating it. Whereas in developing countries about 2 oz (60 g) dietary fibre enters the large bowel daily the amount is usually over ½oz (20 g) in Western countries. If fibre intake were adequate, laxatives would seldom be required.

From this description, you can see that fibre is by no means an insignificant factor in diet. It plays a very important role in digestive processes, and its presence or absence has many repercussions. The following chapters will show in detail its special significance in relation to various common Western diseases and will explain how they may be prevented.

6 DISEASES RELATED TO BOWEL CONTENT

There are three common diseases related to the nature of the content of the bowel: constipation, diverticular disease and appendicitis. There is strong evidence that each is caused or aggravated by hard faecal matter, typical of fibre-depleted diets. You will see in this chapter how all three diseases are linked, and how fibre in the diet can provide protection against them.

Constipation

This common word is used to describe the slow movement of unduly firm content through the large bowel leading to the infrequent passing of small hard stools. Views on constipation vary widely. Most people expect to have a bowel motion at least once a day. Some doctors have said, quite wrongly in my opinion, that it does not matter whether you have two motions a day, or three a week.

Some idea of the magnitude of the problem of constipation in Western countries is underlined by the estimation that over £40 million are spent on laxatives annually in Britain; and over $300 million in the United States, in addition to laxatives prescribed by the medical profession.

The size and consistency of stools and the time taken for food to pass

RIGHT: The average daily stool weights in different communities is directly related and the time taken for food residue to pass along the digestive tract is inversely related to fibre intake. High stool weights and low intestinal transit times are associated with low occurrence of all the diseases.

46

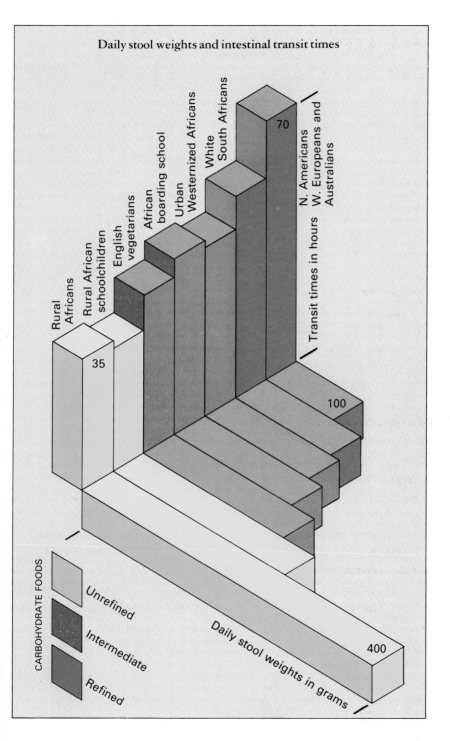

Daily stool weights and intestinal transit times

Rural Africans

Rural African schoolchildren

English vegetarians

African boarding school

Urban Westernized Africans

White South Africans

N. Americans W. Europeans and Australians

Transit times in hours

35

70

100

400

CARBOHYDRATE FOODS

Unrefined

Intermediate

Refined

Daily stool weights in grams

through the digestive tract from mouth to evacuation are the only reliable measurements of bowel behaviour. The amount of stool passed daily in different communities is more closely related to the frequency of the diseases described in chapter three than any other single physiological measurement. Yet there are few aspects of bodily function about which there is more ignorance. Stools are a taboo subject.

As I travel extensively, lecturing all over the world, this lack of knowledge of bowel behaviour is confirmed over and over again. One of my major research projects over the past ten years has been to try to record information on bowel behaviour in different communities in both Third-World and Western countries, and to relate it to disease patterns in these communities.

In rural Africa and other places where most of the food eaten is in the form of minimally-processed, starchy staple carbohydrates such as cereals, legumes (like beans and peas) and root vegetables like potatoes or yams, about 13-17 oz (400-500 g) of soft stool is evacuated by an adult daily. In striking contrast, adults on modern Western diets usually pass on average less than 3–4 oz (80–120 g) of firm stool a day (see page 47).

The average time taken for food residue to pass along the whole of the intestinal tract has been scientifically measured and again the figures are very different. The people being investigated were asked to swallow unabsorbable radio-opaque plastic markers. Stools are then collected and X-rayed. The markers can be readily identified and counted. The time when the markers are swallowed and stools passed is recorded, and the time taken for an agreed proportion of the markers (usually 80 per cent) to pass out in the stools can be estimated. This is known as the intestinal transit time.

This intestinal transit time averages only about one and a half days in rural communities in the Third World. In Western countries this usually takes about three days in young healthy adults. Among the elderly it often takes over two weeks. There is no denying that the populations of Western communities are by world standards extremely constipated. It is becoming increasingly accepted by doctors that this is mainly due to a deficiency of dietary fibre.

Evidence from the past
Fortunately some evidence is still available about the type of stools passed by our ancestors long before the common diseases became such a

48

The Fifth Tribe, are the *Merdæ Sphærulatæ*, *five Balanoides*, the Button formed Excrement ; there are two Species of this Tribe, the firſt are thoſe voided in ſmall, firm, round, diſtinct Balls, Buttons, or Bullets ; the ſecond are thoſe kind of Buttons conglomerate, or joined ſo cloſe and compact together, as to form, at firſt ſight, one large ſolid Excrement, but upon a cloſer Scrutiny they lie *racematim* or *ſpicatim*, like an Ear of *Indian* Wheat, and may as eaſily be ſeparated, if any one wou'd undertake the Work.

I have obſerved theſe Species to flouriſh moſtly about Colleges, Schools, and moſt Places of publick Education.

This facsimile page from *Human Ordure* by Dean Swift describes the stools to be avoided.

major scourge. Dean Jonathan Swift, the author of *Gulliver's Travels*, wrote a little book entitled *Human Ordure*, the old English word for excreta. He gave his name on the title page as 'Dr S. . .t', as if shy to disclose the identity of the author of a book on such a taboo subject. This book was published in Dublin in 1733 at the price of sixpence. In it he classified the different types of stool, found in and around Dublin, into five categories, just as botanists catalogue plant species. The most satisfactory stool, in his opinion, he likened to 'a boy's top reversed'. That is with the flat surface down and the point upwards. Such a stool can easily be found in Third-World countries today. The worst stools were likened to 'balls, buttons or bullets' (see above), an apt description of the small hard stools often passed in Western countries today.

What effect does dietary fibre have on stools?
When diets are rich in dietary fibre the stools passed are usually large in volume, pale in colour, soft in consistency and float in water. The reverse is true of stools associated with fibre-depleted diets. There is little evidence that drinking water or other fluids will have any useful

effect in treating constipation. Without enough fibre, fluid is simply absorbed from the bowel and excreted in the urine.

Some knowledge of the nature of human or pre-human stools has recently been traced back to Paleolithic man. Stools estimated to have been passed over 100,000 years ago were rehydrated and their original weight estimated at about 8 oz (220 g). This is approximately the weight of each stool passed by people in rural communities in the Third World today – who usually pass two motions daily. It might therefore be reasonably assumed that our distant ancestors had bowel behaviour not dissimilar to rural Africans today, and that it is only within the last century or so that Western nations have become generally constipated due to inadequate fibre in the national diets.

Diverticular disease of the colon

In Western countries about one in ten people over the age of forty and one in three over sixty have diverticular disease. Constipation is now recognized as the underlying cause.

Diverticular disease is the development of small, blown-out pouches in the wall of the colon. It was the first disease to be generally accepted throughout the medical profession as resulting from constipation and, therefore, from fibre-depleted diets. This is particularly remarkable as, until recently, diverticular disease had been customarily treated by specifically restricting fibre or 'roughage' in the diet. Roughage was a regrettable term since it suggested that fibre-rich diets resulted in rough bowel content which was irritating the lining of the bowel. This was a misconception, and 'softage' would have been a better designation since fibre ensures soft rather than rough bowel content. Diverticulitis (see above, right), the better known term, denotes inflammation of one or more diverticula. It is only rarely that diverticula become infected. They can however cause much abdominal pain and discomfort, although they often give rise to few symptoms and remain undetected.

How diverticula develop

When the content of the colon is soft and voluminous it can easily be propelled along inside the gut by the rhythmic peristaltic waves of contraction of the muscle in the bowel wall (see page 42). When the content is firm in consistency and reduced in volume, due to excessive

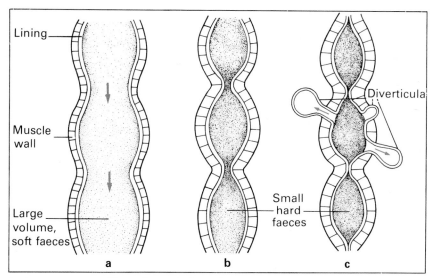

In these cross-sections through the colon:

a On a high-fibre diet the high-volume, soft faecal content is propelled along easily.

b On a low-fibre diet the small, hard faecal content needs extra effort from the muscles in the bowel wall which becomes stronger.

c These increased pressures can eventually force pouches of the lining through the muscle wall. These are the diverticula.

absorption of water, it becomes resistant to onward propulsion and the bowel-wall muscle has to exert much additional effort to ensure its forward movement. To understand how the firmness of faeces increases the effort required for its onward propulsion, compare the ease of pushing a pat of butter along inside a rubber tube with the effort required to squeeze a lump of tar, or any other substance of firm consistency.

To cope with these extra demands the muscle thickens in an attempt to increase its efficiency, and this inevitably results in greatly increased pressures within the bowel. In time, these unnatural pressures can force pouches of the bowel lining out through the wall of the gut. These are the diverticula (see above, right). The blowing out of diverticula can be compared to the way the inner tube of a bicycle wheel can bulge out through a defect in the outer tyre, or the way that clay pushes out between the fingers when the hand holding it is clenched (see overleaf).

Now that the role of fibre is better understood, the idea that a low-fibre diet might benefit this disease has been abandoned. If the

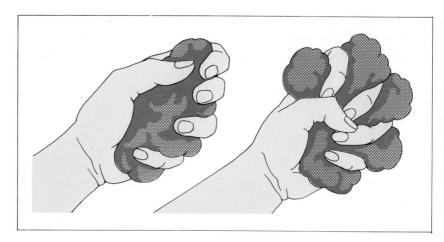

Diverticula develop in the same way as mud held in the hand is forced out between the fingers when the fist is clenched.

small, hard, drier stools associated with constipation lead to diverticula formation, then the aim must be to encourage large, soft, moist stools – a result that can be achieved by eating fibre. As Dr Kenneth Heaton, one of the leaders in research on dietary fibre has so neatly expressed it, the recipe for satisfactory bowel behaviour is 'hard in and soft out', implying that if the food eaten is rich in fibre, the stools evacuated will, as a result, be soft. This aphorism is not entirely true as fibre-rich foods need not necessarily be hard.

This new understanding of the nature of diverticular disease explains its rarity even in Western countries until about sixty years ago; before then the diet of Western countries still contained adequate fibre. This also accounts for the almost total absence of the disease in Third-World countries today where the daily diet is still rich in fibre.

Once a disease has developed, discovering and removing the cause does not get rid of the disease itself and some form of treatment is often necessary. On the other hand, treating a disease without, at the same time, attempting to remove or reduce the factors causing it is like snatching a child out of a fire, treating his burns, and then putting him back in the flames which were responsible for causing his burns in the first place. Eliminating the cause is always better than merely treating the symptoms of a disease. For example, it is better to seal the leak in a pipe than to keep putting buckets underneath to collect the escaping water.

Any treatment of diverticular disease should therefore be accompanied by a change in diet. In almost all British, and in an increasing proportion of American, clinics all patients with diverticular disease of the colon, whether with or without symptons, are put on high-fibre diets. In some hospitals this approach has reduced the proportion of patients requiring surgical treatment by as much as 90 per cent.

Appendicitis

I have already referred to the relationship between appendicitis and economic development, and have emphasized its rarity among traditionally living peoples and its sharply reduced occurrence during wartime food rationing. Appendicitis is rarely found among rural communities in the Third World. When Africans from certain colonial countries were sent to Europe for further training they became, in their new environment, liable to develop appendicitis, which was very rare among them when they were back home. In the Second World War, when African troops insisted they be issued with British Army rations, appendicitis began for the first time to appear among them.

Professor Rendle-Short showed in 1920 the rarity of appendicitis among prisoners in Britain who consumed a coarser diet compared to those outside. A recent study in Wales has shown that people who had consistently eaten brown or wholemeal bread had a lower risk of developing appendicitis than those who had habitually eaten white bread.

What is appendicitis?

The appendix is a blind-ended tube about two inches long opening into the beginning of the large intestine, known as the caecum (see overleaf).

Appendicitis is an inflammation of the appendix. The suffix 'itis' added to the name of any organ denotes inflammation. For example tonsillitis, diverticulitis, gastritis and hepatitis refer to inflamation of the tonsils, diverticula, the bowel, the stomach and the liver respectively. But in the case of appendicitis bacterial invasion is not the start of the trouble. Infection comes after the blocking of the cavity of the appendix.

What causes this blockage? How can we account for the enormous variation in the occurrence of appendicitis round the world? Why is it commoner among the young than older people? Why does it appear to be more common during certain virus infections? These are the questions that need to be answered.

Often a small hard lump of faecal matter, about the size of a pea, is found causing the blockage (see below). This exists only in the presence of the firmer faeces that are associated with fibre-depleted diets. When this type of obstruction has not occurred it has been suggested that the cause may be excessive muscular contraction. This could occur through the exaggerated efforts of the muscle in the appendix wall to push out a firm faecal particle from the narrow cavity into the colon. Such muscle spasm can, in the presence of firm faecal content, close off the much wider cavity of the appendix.

The changes that lead to obstruction of the inside of the appendix will depend not only on the softness or hardness of the contents of the colon but also on the width of the appendix cavity. We have so far considered the former but not the latter. Until the age of about twenty, the

A small hard particle of faeces blocks the appendix.

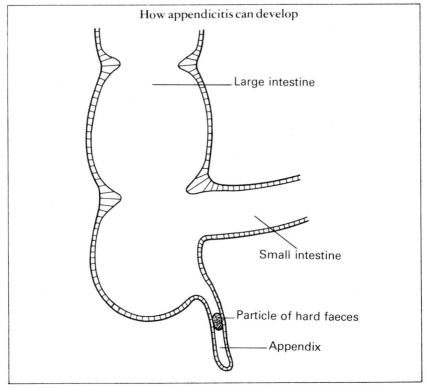

How appendicitis can develop

Large intestine

Small intestine

Particle of hard faeces

Appendix

lymphoid tissue (which is the same kind of tissue that is found in lymph glands and tonsils), takes up much space in the wall of the appendix thus narrowing the cavity. After that time it decreases in amount as the person grows older. This lymphoid tissue swells when it becomes infected and so further narrows the free cavity inside the appendix and makes it more likely to get blocked. This could explain not only the increased frequency of appendicitis among young people, but also why appendicitis sometimes occurs after virus infections which result in swelling of the lymphoid tissue.

Once appendicitis has developed it needs urgent treatment. Although relatively mild cases may get better after treatment with antibiotic drugs, surgical removal of the appendix is usually the treatment of choice. If the patient is not seen until the disease has been present for several days the infection may have already spread beyond the appendix to form an abscess. Such an abscess may subside after treatment with antibiotics or it may require surgical drainage. In either case it is usually advised that the appendix be removed after the inflammation has subsided.

In different communities there is an inverse relationship between fibre intake and the frequency of operations for the removal of the appendix. Keeping bowel content soft seems to provide the best safeguard against the development of appendicitis. Sufficient fibre in the diet will do this. We can do nothing to alter the nature or amount of the lymphoid tissue in our appendices to prevent them swelling up. We *can* alter the consistency of our bowel content by the simple dietary changes recommended in chapter twelve.

Lack of dietary fibre is the only adequate explanation of the cause of appendicitis, given our present knowledge, and it is consistent with the clinical, pathological and epidemiological features of the disease. Here again, prevention seems to depend on diet. The three diseases discussed in this chapter are all related to hard bowel content. Of course it is the ability of fibre to retain water and so ensure larger, softer stools that makes it a suitable remedy. The next chapter is also related to bowel content, but more specifically to the abdominal straining necessary to passing hard stools. As will be seen, alterations in bowel content and behaviour caused by fibre-depleted diets can lead to other associated diseases.

7 DISEASES RELATED TO ABDOMINAL STRAINING

The three diseases to be described in this chapter: hiatus hernia, varicose veins and piles have been attributed in part to increased pressures within the muscle walls that surround the abdomen as a result of straining to evacuate stools. Once more, the problem appears to be due to excess removal of water from the contents of the bowel, so that stools are small and hard and therefore difficult to evacuate.

Defaecation

This is the technical word for evacuating stools. The presence of firm, small-volume content in the rectum, the last portion of the intestine, has an important significance in connection with defaecation. It makes it necessary to forcibly contract the muscles of the abdominal wall to pass a stool. A resistant, unyielding mass of firm faecal matter is obviously more difficult to force through the anal canal, the name given to the back passage (the last inch or so of the intestinal tract) than a soft pliable mass. The anal canal is far narrower than the bowel above it and is surrounded by a muscle called a sphincter. When this muscle is contracted it closes the passage off in the same way that a rubber tube can be closed by tying a piece of string tightly around it. This sphincter normally remains contracted to prevent bowel content escaping, but relaxes when a stool is being passed. It can thus be compared to a tap or faucet which allows water to pass through it only when turned on.

There is another mechanism concerned with stool evacuation. Once the rectum has filled up sufficiently, the stretching of the muscle in its wall triggers a mechanism that makes this muscle contract and lets you feel you want to evacuate some stools. This contraction squeezes the faeces out of the rectum rather like the way that squeezing a tube of toothpaste forces out its contents, and at the same time the sphincter opens to let the stool pass through.

Difficulties with defaecation

The rectum has to contain about 7 oz (200 g) of stool to initiate an adequate emptying response by the muscle in its wall. On modern, Western fibre-depleted diets it is rare to have this amount of faeces in the rectum, so adequate squeezing of the muscle in the bowel wall does not occur, and consequently the muscles in the wall of the abdomen have to work more to empty the firm contents of the bowel (page 51). This straining at stool is a characteristic feature of our Western way of life.

There is another factor that may hinder the efficiency with which we empty our bowels. The usual way to pass a stool, even in Western countries until a century ago and still today in most of the world, was to squat. In this position, the thighs are pressed against the abdominal wall and this is believed to assist stool evacuation. Modern man prefers to sit, for he knows that he will probably have to wait a long time before stool is passed. Straining greatly raises the pressure within the abdominal cavity. Some of the results of this straining, causing raised abdominal pressures, will now be considered.

Hiatus hernia

This is the name given to a condition in which the top of the stomach is pushed upwards out of the abdomen and into the thoracic cavity, the part of the body above the diaphragm, which is a sheet of muscle separating the abdomen from the thorax (page 42). The thorax contains the heart and lungs and normally the oesophagus or gullet joins the stomach just below the diaphragm.

Any upward displacement of the stomach through the hole in the diaphragm through which the oesophagus passes is known as a hiatus hernia (see overleaf). In North America this condition can be found in about one in five middle-aged adults by X-ray examination of their stomach, following the swallowing of a radio-opaque meal containing

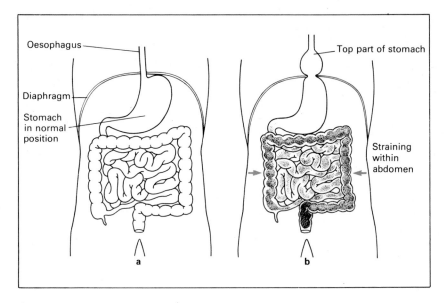

Oesophagus

Top part of stomach

Diaphragm

Stomach in normal position

Straining within abdomen

a

b

Pressures within the abdomen raised when straining to evacuate hard faeces from the rectum can force the top of the stomach up through the hole in the diaphragm **b** through which the oesophagus passes. This is considered an important cause of hiatus hernia.

barium. Although in the majority of cases it is not associated with any symptoms it is a common cause of heartburn. Both hiatus hernia and heartburn are rare in Third-World communities.

A protrusion of the stomach up through the diaphragm must either be caused by a push from below, a pull up from above, or a combination of both. The most likely cause is understandably reckoned to be a push from below, so what is this push likely to be?

If a hole is cut in the wall of a tennis ball (right, above) and it is then filled with water and squeezed, the water will be forced out through the hole (right, below). The abdominal cavity can be compared to a tennis ball. There is a hole in its wall down through which the gullet passes to join the stomach. When the ball is squeezed the abdominal muscles forcibly contract, as in straining at stool. The upper end of the stomach is then squeezed up out of the abdomen rather like the water coming out of a tennis ball. This is the only explanation for the cause of hiatus hernia that is consistent with the distribution of the disease, although it cannot yet be considered a proven cause.

Recent studies have shown that pressures within the abdominal

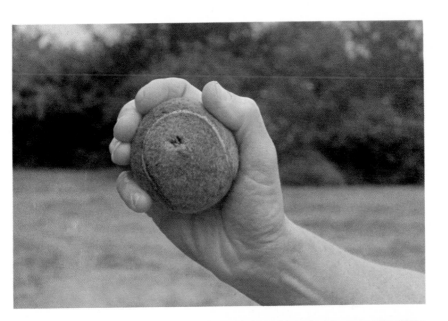

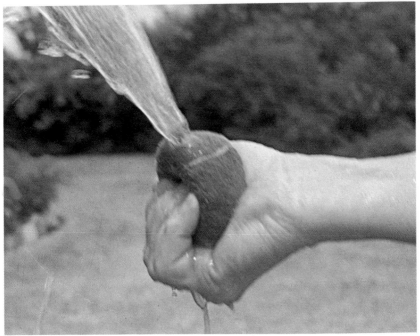

The development of a hiatus hernia can be compared to the way water can be squeezed through a hole in a tennis ball.

cavity rise to over 75 in (190 cm) of water when straining to pass stool, whereas those in the thoracic cavity rise to only 25 in (67 cm) of water. This shows that the pressures below the diaphragm are much greater than those above. The scientists who did these studies concluded that their findings were consistent with the hypothesis that straining at stool was an important factor in the causation of hiatus hernia.

Hiatus hernia is associated not only in its geographical distribution, but also in individual patients, with both diverticular disease and gallstones. This suggests that all three diseases share some common cause. Once again, our way of life and, specifically, our fibre-depleted diet largely seem to be responsible.

Heartburn is caused by acid stomach juices entering the lower end of the gullet. When the junction between the gullet and the stomach is in its normal position below the diaphragm the muscle round the lower end of the gullet prevents the stomach contents flowing back up. When the stomach has been pushed up into the thorax the closure of the lower end of the gullet (which usually acts like a valve, squeezing to shut itself off) becomes less efficient, allowing acid stomach contents to enter it.

Heartburn is often treated with alkalis to neutralize the acid juices that irritate the lining of the gullet. Raising the head of the bed at night will help to minimize the entry of gastric juices into the gullet. In some patients with persistent pain, surgery is sometimes advised to repair the defect and restore the upper end of the stomach to its normal position below the diaphragm. The addition of fibre in the diet would help reduce the straining associated with hiatus hernia and might avoid the need for surgery.

Varicose veins

Veins are said to be varicose when they are tortuous and swollen. The occasional varicose veins that result from blockage of the deep leg veins by blood clots will not be considered here.

Blood from the legs is returned to the heart through the veins. To prevent blood flowing back down the legs due to gravity instead of up to the heart, the veins have a series of valves which permit blood to flow towards the heart but in the opposite direction. The flow of blood is moved along by muscle contraction around the deep veins; this contraction squeezes the veins and thus pushes the blood in one direction only

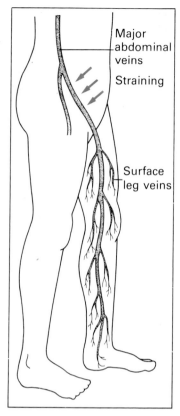

Major abdominal veins

Straining

Surface leg veins

The valves in the veins ensure that blood flows back up to the heart.

(see left). The mechanism is similar to a pump forcing water uphill. The pump pushes the water up and valves prevent its return.

Veins susceptible to swelling and distortion lie under the skin near the surface of the legs, and so have less support around them than the deeper veins which are surrounded by muscles. Varicosities develop when the valves become defective so that they no longer protect the veins below them from the backward flow of blood from above (see overleaf).

Are varicose veins caused by some inherent weakness in the vein walls, or their valves? There is certainly no evidence to support this suggestion. Consequently varicose veins must be caused by damage to the veins. The most likely reason why veins become incompetent is that abdominal straining forces blood back down the leg veins, stretching then so that the valves cannot function properly. The unsupported weight of blood then progressively distorts the veins.

The evidence for an environmental factor

People in Western nations are affected much more by varicose veins than those in rural communities in developing countries. In Western countries varicose veins are more common among women than men, but not to the extent that hospital attendances would indicate, as women are more likely to seek treatment for cosmetic reasons. Varicose veins do not usually give rise to pain or disability.

In developing countries they are often more frequently found among men. In poorer countries with high birth rates varicose veins are far less common than in more affluent countries with much lower birth rates.

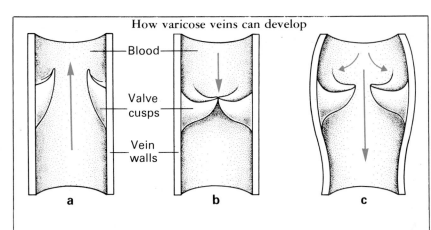

How varicose veins can develop

Blood
Valve cusps
Vein walls

a   b   c

a   The valves ensure that blood flows only back up to the heart.

b   They prevent backflow as the valve cusps meet each other and close the vein.

c   Blood forced back down the veins over a period, stretches the walls so that the valves are unable to meet.

These observations make it no longer possible to assume that pregnancy, or the constrictive clothing once worn by women, are primary causes of varicose veins.

Results of epidemiological studies also refute the widely held view that hereditary factors are a major cause. A survey of the extent of varicose veins among populations in the Pacific showed that they were more closely related to Western culture than to any other factor. The problem was rarest in the islands whose traditional culture had been least changed, and most common among those most influenced by the Western way of life. The occurrence of varicose veins among New Zealand Maori women is higher than among white New Zealanders. Islands with an intermediate culture, such as the Cook Islands in the Pacific, partly traditional and partly Western, have an intermediate occurrence of varicose veins.

Varicose veins are just as common today among black Americans as whites. In rural Africa varicose veins are relatively rare everywhere. As black Americans originally came from Africa this shows that the cause of their varicose veins could hardly be genetic, otherwise they would still be less prone to develop them. Genetic susceptibility probably does play a secondary role, but when diseases run in families it does not necessarily have to be due to hereditary factors. It could equally well be because families tend to have the same dietary and other habits.

Some people have suggested that standing all day increases the likelihood of getting varicose veins as this might place excessive pressure on the leg veins. But if this is so, why do the trishaw men mentioned on page 27 suffer more from the problem than barbers? Both, after all, are on their feet all day. The answer, surely, must be that the former are straining as they pull their modern versions of rickshaws, while the latter are merely standing still. Although the main reason for abdominal straining is to assist the evacuation of firm faecal mass from the bowel, any persistent straining activity such as trishaw riding can have a similar effect.

It might be argued that all heavy physical work involves some contraction of abdominal muscles. It has been shown though that such enormously strenuous exercise as weight-lifting raises pressures within the abdomen to a lesser extent than does straining at stool.

This increased abdominal pressure caused by straining to pass small firm stools has been singled out as a major cause of hiatus hernia and varicose veins. It also seems likely that varicose veins share a common cause with diverticular disease. Both diseases occur most often in the same communities, and patients with diverticular disease are more likely to have varicose veins than people without this disease. Once more, hard faeces set up a chain of events far removed from mere constipation.

Once varicose veins have developed, removing their cause will not undo the harm already done. Varicose veins often require no treatment except for cosmetic reasons. Those that do need treatment can often be improved with injections of a fluid that sticks the walls together, thus blocking the cavity and preventing the backward flow of blood. More severe cases may be dealt with by ligatures that tie off the veins and so cut off the blood supply. Surgical removal of part of the diseased vein may be necessary.

Varicose veins are rare among people under the age of twenty but become progressively more common with increasing age. This suggests that the cause lies in a progressive and cumulative effect of some environmental factor operating over a long period of time. Animals do not suffer from varicose veins, which indicates that the basic cause must be something in the way of life peculiar to human beings. The evidence thus suggests that inadequate fibre in our diet is an important cause of varicose veins.

Piles (haemorrhoids)

I have already mentioned that haemorrhoids, often referred to as piles, are found everywhere. They are, however, much more common in Western countries than among people living in the Third World. Before looking at the cause of piles it is necessary to consider what they are and how they can occur. True piles must be distinguished from little tender painful swellings near the anal margin referred to as 'external piles', which are clots of blood caused by the rupture of small veins under the skin. They must also be distinguished from harmless tags of skin which are a common occurrence round the anal margin.

Until recently it has always been assumed that piles are varicosities of the veins in the anal canal analogous to varicose veins in the legs, but recent research has suggested that this is not in fact the case. It now

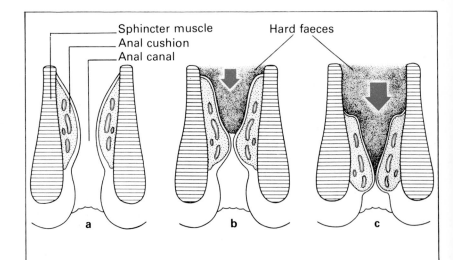

a   The anal cushions in their normal position to prevent escape of faeces.
b   The passage of hard faeces forces them down.
c   Eventually piles occur.

seems that piles are a downward prolapse of normal cushions full of blood vessels that surround the upper end of the anal canal to help prevent the escape of faeces (see below). These cushions are present from birth. When they are swollen and are pushed down through the anal canal they are called piles.

How piles occur

What is it that makes the anal cushions become swollen and pushes them down the anal canal? In the first place they become engorged with blood and swollen as a result of abdominal straining. So long as faecal matter is soft, and straining is not necessary, the soft content comes out easily through the anal canal. When the stool is hard the straining that is necessary for its evacuation forces blood into the cushions which swell up as a result. The expulsion of the hard faecal mass requires further straining and the shearing stress of its passage, repeated many times along the anal canal, gradually pushes the cushions down away from their natural position towards the anal margin (see left, below).

It seems likely that this is the way piles are caused. This explanation was first given by the British surgeon, Hamish Thomson, and is more closely consistent with all available evidence than any other theory. Constipation is a fundamental underlying cause. There are almost certainly other causes not yet identified, but a high proportion of patients suffering from piles will require no further treatment once they have switched to a high-fibre diet and as a result produce soft stools that can be passed with minimal straining. Many surgical clinics are now finding that, as in the case of diverticular disease, the proportion of patients with piles requiring surgical treatment is greatly reduced once their diet has been changed. Some patients will, however, require simple surgical procedures and in a few the piles will need to be surgically removed. Whatever the treatment, a diet rich in fibre is the best way to guard against recurrence of the problem.

The three diseases discussed in this chapter – hiatus hernia, varicose veins and piles – are shown to have one cause in common. If they are all due in part to abdominal straining because of hard, small stools, a very simple way to reduce their prevalence would be, quite simply, to eat more fibre. The amounts of fibre in various foods and the recommended daily intake are discussed in chapters twelve and thirteen.

8 THE BACKGROUND TO LARGE BOWEL CANCER

Where it occurs and why

Cancer of the large bowel is another disease related to bowel behaviour and content. It is also the most serious of those so far discussed. Cancer of the large bowel affects both the colon and rectum. In North America, northern Europe and Australasia it is the commonest cause of death from cancer, apart from lung cancer caused by smoking.

Tumours of the colon and of the rectum have their highest and their lowest frequencies in the same communities. The relative proportions of tumours developing in the colon and the rectum vary, however, in different communities; this suggests that some causes specifically affect either the colon or the rectum in addition to any shared cause affecting both. The frequency of large bowel cancer (also referred to as large intestine and colo-rectal cancer) is more closely related to economic development and a Western way of life than any other form of cancer.

The geographical distribution of large bowel cancer is almost identical to that of non-malignant tumours referred to as polyps. These are present in nearly 20 per cent of adults in Western countries but usually cause no trouble and remain unrecognized. Many pathologists believe, with good evidence, that most cancers of the bowel develop from a pre-existing polyp. It must, however, be emphasized that only a very small proportion of polyps ever turn into a cancer, but the more polyps in the bowel the greater the risk that one may become maligant.

In countries where the prevalence of large bowel cancer is low, polyps of the bowel are rare; this includes most of Asia and the whole of Africa. In Africa, polyps are extremely rare. For instance, only six patients with polyps were detected over a period of thirteen years in a South African hospital with over 2000 beds and high medical standards.

As the distribution of both polyps and malignant tumours is almost identical it is generally agreed that they have similar or closely linked causes and that these causes are almost certainly found in the food that is eaten. This does not mean that it is poisonous, or contains cancer-inducing substances, but that in the large intestine it can promote the formation of cancer-inducing substances, known as carcinogens, probably through bacterial activity.

Despite the overall size, the membrane lining of the large bowel is well over 100 times *smaller* than the lining of the small bowel. In the latter, the lining is folded up and down like a pleated skirt, so that its total surface area is very much more extensive than is apparent when examining the inside of the bowel. This folding does not apply to the large bowel and it is why the total surface area of the small intestine is so much greater than the large intestine.

On the other hand both benign and malignant tumours occur over 100 times more frequently in the large than in the small intestine. This means that, relative to surface area, tumours are at least 10,000 times more common in the large intestine. What does this unequal distribution of tumours in the intestine suggest? Even if the lining of the large bowel is somehow more prone to tumour development, this enormous discrepancy strongly suggests that the carcinogens responsible are actually formed in the colon rather than transmitted to it through the small intestine after being swallowed in the food.

Diets that appear perfectly alright in other respects may lead to processes occurring within the gut that could increase the production, or the concentration of, carcinogens. It may take fifty or more years for cancer to occur. In order to discover what factors in diet might cause large bowel cancer let us look at different communities which have unusually low or high incidences of this disease.

Although bowel cancer is more common in richer than in poorer countries, some communities within the richer group may be less affected than the group as a whole. For example, Seventh Day Adventists, who are predominently vegetarians, have a diet richer in fibre and lower in animal fat than other Americans and suffer from about one third less bowel cancer. The same applies to Mormons who are not vegetarians and who have a fat intake comparable to other Americans.

(Incidentally, both of these religious denominations have an exceedingly low frequency of lung cancer because, among both of them, smoking is justifiably condemned.)

The life-style of Finns is similar to that of Danes. Yet Copenhagen Danes have been shown to have four times more colon cancer than rural Finns. New Yorkers also get about four times more colon cancer than rural Finns and roughly the same amount as the Danes. All these people have comparable fat intakes but the Finns eat nearly twice as much fibre, largely of cereal origin, and pass more than twice as much stool.

Colon cancer appears to be more common in the Argentine, where a higher proportion of animal fat is eaten in the diet, than in other countries in South America. It becomes more common among Eskimos who abandon their traditional way of life and adopt an American way of life. Possible causes of these staggering differences will be discussed later in the chapter.

Changes following emigration

Many communities have increased their risk of developing bowel cancer after emigrating to another country where it is more common. As they adopt the way of life of their new country, including its diet, the disease gradually becomes just as common among the immigrants as in the population of the host country. For example, we may assume that the slaves brought to North America over 200 years ago had a rate of bowel cancer at least as low as that of rural Africans today. Forty or fifty years ago black Americans had more of this disease than rural Africans have even today, but they were still much less affected than white Americans. Yet both groups now have approximately the same chance of suffering from this type of cancer (see page 29).

There is a progressive increase in the liability of black Americans to develop this form of cancer when they conform to the pattern of life associated with modern society — particularly as they adopt the diet and customs of white Americans. Some people might argue that this change in disease pattern might be accounted for by inter-marriage between blacks and whites but this could not explain such dramatic changes within little more than a generation. The Jews who emigrated from the Yemen, North Africa and from parts of the USSR to Israel just after it had been established provide another example. Not only is large bowel cancer much more common among their descendants, but so are other characteristically Western diseases such as diabetes and coronary heart disease.

The Japanese who emigrated to Hawaii and California and adopted an American way of life provide us with one of the most striking examples ever observed of changes in disease patterns following changes in dietary customs. Until the Second World War large bowel cancer was uncommon in Japan, whereas stomach cancer was more common there than anywhere else in the world. Within a generation, Japanese emigrants to the United States had a risk of developing large bowel cancer almost equal to that of other Americans. On the other hand, their risk of developing stomach cancer fell (see page 30).

What are the causes?
So what changes in diet can account for these contrasts in the frequency of bowel cancer?

When discussing dietary changes in chapter four it was emphasized that the proportions of calories in the diet provided by fat and carbohydrate are always inversely related. When fat is increased then carbohydrate is decreased and vice versa. It was also shown that fat and fibre are inversely related to one another to an even greater extent, so that diets high in fibre and low in fat are characteristic of the rural communities in the Third World among whom bowel cancer is rare. In contrast diets high in fat and low in fibre characterize affluent Western communities in which the risk of developing bowel cancer is high. The proportion of animal protein in the diet is usually directly related to fat and inversely related to fibre, and is consequently higher in communities with a high bowel cancer risk.

Evidence currently available strongly suggests that excessive fat in the diet increases the risk of developing large bowel cancer and that fibre provides protection against it. A high animal protein content in the diet of communities that eat a lot of meat, such as those in Argentina, has also been blamed, but the evidence is less convincing than it is for fat. It is regrettable that high-fat and low-fibre diets have been viewed as 'either-or' hypotheses in attempting to explain the cause of large bowel cancer, whereas it seems much more likely that they are 'both-and' explanations. Fat may well be a cause of, while fibre may provide protection against, bowel cancer as in the case of the other diseases being discussed.

The type and number of bacteria in the colon are influenced by the food eaten. These bacteria can act on bile salts or other ingredients of the contents of the colon and convert them into substances that are chemically very similar to known carcinogens (meaning any cancer-causing substances). Fat in the diet increases the amount of bile salts found in the colon on which bacteria act. And if less fat is eaten there will be less bile salts to convert to carcinogens. If carcinogens are diluted in a large faecal volume and carried quicly through the large bowel (as happens with fibre-rich diets), they will be less dangerous than when concentrated in a small faecal volume and delayed in the gut (as happens with fibre-depleted diets). Bowel cancer is invariably rare in communities passing large stools, and stool volume is always small in communities with a high frequency of bowel cancer.

The benefits of fibre and dangers of fat

Support for the protection provided by a high-fibre, low-fat diet is provided by the various communities described earlier. The Seventh Day Adventists eat more fibre and less fat than average Americans and have less bowel cancer risk. Mormons apparently eat as much fat as other Americans but probably eat more cereal fibre as it is a common practice among them to grind their own wheat at home and then make wholemeal bread. The fibre may be protective and could help to neutralize the effect of the large amount of fat in the Mormon diet.

American slaves presumably ate a fibre-rich carbohydrate diet that was also low in fat, comparable to that of rural African villagers today. Forty or fifty years ago the diet of black Americans in the southern States was largely fibre-rich corn meal (maize) and other carbohydrates, with less fat than was available to whites. Their intake of fat and fibre was intermediate between that of Africans and white Americans. Today black and white Americans eat the same diet with the same fat and fibre content and the incidence of bowel cancer is similar for both.

The Jews in the Yemen ate much unrefined wholemeal bread and consequently had a fibre-rich diet, but after emigrating to Israel the fibre content decreased while the fat, sugar and animal protein content increased. The incidence of bowel cancer and of other diseases followed suit.

The Japanese used to eat more cereals in the form of rice and millet and less fat than other industrialized nations, but their pattern of diet is changing. Those that emigrated to the United States and adopted an American way of life have increased their intake of fat and animal protein and decreased the amount of fibre they eat. As we have seen their level of bowel cancer has also increased.

A summary of large bowel cancer

Diet almost definitely controls the pattern of bacteria in the gut, but it is still not certain which component of diet is most responsible for these changes. Various bacteria that are more common in stools from people in Western than in Third-World countries have the ability to change normal bowel content, such as bile salts, into substances that could be cancer-causing.

While fat in the diet increases the amount of bile salts on which the bacteria act, fibre dilutes them and, for reasons not yet understood, reduces bacterial activity. Any carcinogens formed in the faeces will also be diluted if the faeces are of large volume; the action of carcinogens is thereby reduced. Within large-volume faeces, associated with high-fibre diets, these carcinogens will be moved along the bowel more quickly and therefore have less prolonged contact with the lining of the gut in which the cancer forms, than in the case of slowly moving small-volume faeces.

The geographical distribution of large bowel cancer points strongly to changes in the pattern of diet as the cause of the disease. The critical factor seems to be a combination of low consumption of fibre and high consumption of fats. In the next chapter we will look at two of the most common diseases in Western countries.

9 BIOCHEMICAL CHANGES: CORONARY HEART DISEASE AND GALLSTONES

Coronary heart disease and gallstones seem at face value to be very different from each other, with no obvious connection between them. In fact, both diseases are linked to a substance called cholesterol. In the case of coronary heart disease cholesterol contributes to a silting-up of the arteries. It is also the main constituent of gallstones.

How fibre may protect against coronary heart disease is still uncertain. Fibre definitely reduces absorption of cholesterol in the diet and increases elimination in the stools of bile acids which are derived from it. A high-fibre diet also tends to be a low-fat diet and too much animal fat is thought to increase cholesterol levels in the blood. In this chapter I will try to summarize some of the evidence supporting the argument that fibre in the diet provides protection against both coronary heart disease and gallstones. Other protective and hazardous factors will also be discussed.

Coronary heart disease

This is a disease of the coronary arteries that supply blood to the heart muscle. If these arteries are severely narrowed as a result of a silting-up process insufficient blood gets to the heart muscle to enable it to work normally. This results in severe chest pain known as angina. If blood clots in one of the narrowed arteries, called the coronary arteries, supplying blood to the heart muscle, part of the heart muscle is almost totally deprived of blood and may consequently die. This is what happens when someone has a heart attack. If the heart muscle is able to get some, but not enough, blood, the patient may show signs of heart failure.

This silting-up and narrowing of the arteries all over the body happens gradually as we get older and is called atherosclerosis. Everyone in Western countries gets this disease to a certain extent – so much so that it has been said, with some accuracy, that a man is as old as his arteries (overleaf). Atherosclerosis often occurs first in the large artery, called the aorta, that runs down the back of the chest and abdomen. Even Africans, who still get extremely little coronary heart disease, often have considerable atherosclerosis of the aorta. Among Africans atherosclerosis starts at a later age and rarely spreads to the coronary arteries. Even when it does spread the disease is less severe.

It is possible that very small clots often occur in our coronary arteries but these are broken down and got rid of by the natural protective action of the blood. In Africans any blood clots are broken down more quickly than in Western people – for reasons not yet understood. Because of this and because their arteries are wider coronary thrombosis is still rare in Africans, especially those living in rural areas.

Who gets coronary heart disease?
This disease is the commonest cause of death in the Western world. It is commoner among men than women. One man in four dies from it. As already mentioned, it is very rare in rural Africa or indeed wherever people work hard and have a simple, natural diet. It is certainly very rare in China except in a few large cities and is uncommon in rural India. In Indian cities, however, it may, at least in the upper social class, be almost as common as in Western countries.

There is far less coronary heart disease in the country areas of southern and eastern Europe than in northern and western Europe. Italians who had emigrated to Australia developed more coronary heart disease than those who stayed in Italy. In one town American Italians, who had retained their traditional food habits, were shown to suffer less from coronary heart disease than other Americans. Coronary heart disease increases with emigration from regions where a traditional way of life is maintained to those where a more affluent life-style is customary.

The Jews who emigrated to Israel from the then poorer Middle Eastern countries of Iraq, Iran and the Yemen had low coronary heart disease death rates on arrival in Israel. Subsequently this rate increased

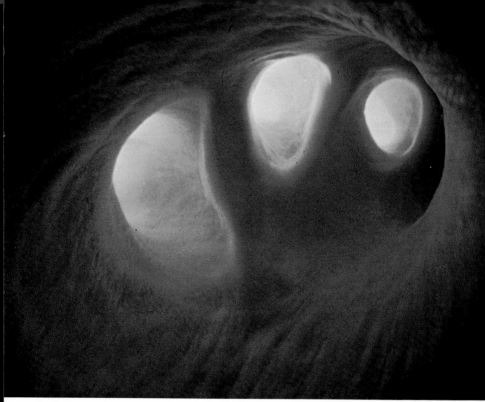

ABOVE: This one-year-old child's coronary artery is absolutely clear.

BELOW: A sixty-year-old man's, silted-up by atherosclerosis.

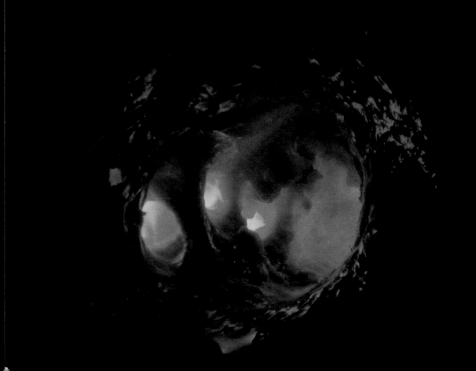

greatly and eventually equalled that of those born in Israel. These examples show that environmental rather than genetic factors are responsible. Undoubtedly there has been a great increase of coronary heart disease deaths in all affluent Western countries during the present century. It has in fact been truthfully called the greatest epidemic mankind has ever known.

Coronary heart disease was first clearly recognized in the 1920s after the electrocardiogram came into general use. Sir William Osler, of Baltimore in the United States and later of Oxford, England, one of the greatest physicians of all time, stated in 1920 that most doctors would see at least one patient suffering from angina during their career but that few medical students would see a case during their medical training. Since 1920 this disease has changed in Western countries from being a rare occurrence to being the commonest cause of death.

It has been insinuated that most of these diseases have not been recorded in Third-World countries because of a lack of proper diagnostic facilities. In the 600-bed teaching hospital in which I worked in Uganda meticulous autopsies were performed on 85 per cent of all patients who died. Less than one case of coronary heart disease was found each year among the 98 per cent of patients who were Africans.

What are the risk factors?
There has been a great deal of research to try to establish why some people and not others get coronary heart disease. In spite of much work many aspects of the disease still remain a puzzle. It has been clearly established, however, that there are certain risk factors. The most important of these are:

Smoking, particularly cigarette smoking, considerably increases the risk of developing coronary heart disease. There is, however, little understanding of why heavy cigarette smoking has this effect.

Foods containing much fat, especially animal fats All countries in which the disease is common are relatively affluent and in them the level of fat consumption is high. Fat, which is present in the substance that silts up the arteries, is transported in the blood in cholesterol. In all countries in which coronary heart disease is common the blood contains high levels of cholesterol. Where the disease is rare cholesterol levels in the blood are low. While this relationship between blood cholesterol levels and the risk of coronary heart disease is true of communities, it is not necessarily true for individuals. A person who lives, say, in the United States and has a low blood cholesterol level cannot be certain he will never have a heart attack. Similarly, many men with high blood cholesterol levels never develop coronary heart disease. It is certain though that people who eat a lot of fat tend to have high blood cholesterol levels and that, if they reduce the fat in their diet, their blood cholesterol levels fall. What is not certain is whether the risk of the disease has been reduced as the blood cholesterol levels fall. The weight of current evidence suggests that excessive intake of fat, and of animal fat in particular, increases the risk of developing coronary heart disease because of the connection with raised cholesterol levels. But it must be added that this is disputed by some authorities.

Salty foods Salt is considered a risk by some doctors because it may be linked with high blood pressure (called hypertension).

Certainly it is a fact that salt consumption is epidemiologically related to the world-wide distribution of high blood pressure, which significantly increases the risk of developing coronary heart disease. Inhabitants of the north island of Japan have the highest consumption of salt in the world, about 1 oz (30 g) each day, and the highest evidence of high blood pressure. In contrast, communities with minimal salt intake, less than $\frac{1}{4}$ oz (5 g) each day, such as parts of New Guinea, have almost no high blood pressure. People living in Western countries consuming about $\frac{1}{2}$ oz (15 g) of salt each day have an intermediate frequency of high blood pressure.

Diabetes and obesity are both linked with an increased risk of developing coronary heart disease. The risk is certainly apparent among diabetic patients. This could be because diabetes itself increases the risk or, alternatively, it might be that both diseases are related because they are caused by the same common factor (see pages 82-88). High blood pressure increases the risk. Once again a curious fact has been observed. Africans who develop high blood pressure rarely develop coronary heart disease, so it seems as if some protective factor is safeguarding them. This may be their diet, though their high degree of physical exercise could also protect them.

Fat people are more likely to develop coronary heart disease than those who are slim. This may not necessarily mean that obesity causes coronary heart disease. It may be that the two diseases are associated because they share common causes as emphasized in chapter one. Even overweight Africans, and there are many of them nowadays particularly in urban areas, rarely develop coronary heart disease.

Other risk factors have been blamed. Some doctors have blamed sugar but most do not consider it a major risk factor. Sugar consumption is very high in certain Latin American countries where coronary heart disease is still uncommon.

Stress has often been blamed as a cause of heart attack. It is, however, fallacious to reckon that stress is a prerogative of Western man and there is no good evidence that it causes the disease. Until the last few years coronary heart disease death rates have been rising almost every year in Britain, at least since the 1920s, but they fell for a few years during the Second World War when nightly bombing must have increased stress. These were the years in which imposed food rationing altered the national diet. Death rates due to heart disease are now beginning to fall in North America and to level out in Britain. This is possibly the result of a reduction in cigarette smoking and of some lowering of the intake of animal fats.

What are the protective factors?
Like the scales mentioned on page 18, coronary heart disease depends on an imbalance between risk factors and protective factors. We have looked at the risk factors, and will now consider what can provide protection.

Exercise Regular and prolonged physical exercise is considered by many doctors to be a protective factor. This increases the demands of the muscles (which includes the heart) for oxygen. Consequently the arteries dilate and carry more blood to the heart and other muscles. People who exercise regularly or have to walk long distances to work may acquire protection.

How diet can protect against heart disease There is no doubt that Third-world diets are associated with a low prevalence of Western-type diseases but the reason for this is not entirely clear. Although the low consumption of fat appears to be part of the answer few would claim that it provides the entire solution.

A United States Senate Committee (known as the McGovern Committee), took more evidence on coronary heart disease than on any other disease. Its report provided guidelines for diet that included recommendations that more wholegrain foods, less animal fat and sugar, and also less butter, eggs and salt should be eaten. The McGovern Committee findings will be described in greater detail in chapter twelve.

Certain types of fibre may also provide protection against coronary heart disease. For instance, when a project researching into the cause of this disease carefully examined a group of men in London, recording their way of life and following their subsequent history for twenty years or until they died, the strongest risk factor for coronary heart disease was found to be smoking and the strongest protective factor, the intake of cereal fibre. Fruit and vegetable fibre provided no protection.

Dr Risteárd Mulcahy's companion title in this series *Beat Heart Disease!* provides more information about the risk and preventive factors for coronary heart disease.

Gallstones

The gall-bladder is a sac attached to the tube that carries the bile, which is formed in the liver, to the first part of the intestine, known as the duodenum. While the bile is in this pouch it loses some of its water and becomes more concentrated than it was when formed in the liver. The situation is similar to that in which bowel content loses water and becomes more concentrated during its relatively slow passage through the large intestine. The gall-bladder stores bile for the times when it is needed, that is for the digestion of fatty foods. After meals it contracts to empty its content into the duodenum where it joins the food leaving the stomach and helps in its digestion (right, above).

Different types of stone can form in the gall-bladder, but by far the most common variety consists largely of cholesterol, and this is the variety that will be discussed here. Gallstones most frequently cause trouble by blocking either the duct between the gall-bladder and the main bile channel from the liver to the duodenum, or by actually blocking the main channel itself. The former causes severe pain due to the efforts of the muscles in the wall of the gall-bladder to empty its content which is blocked by the stone. The latter, main duct obstruction (right, above), is much more serious as it prevents bile leaving the

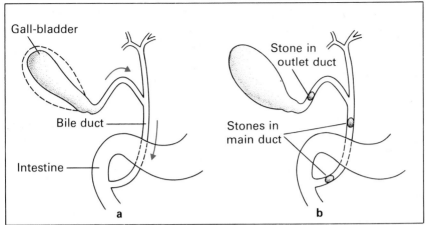

Gall-bladder

Bile duct

Intestine

a

Stone in outlet duct

Stones in main duct

b

a As the gall-bladder contracts bile is squeezed into the intestine to help digestion.

b A stone can block the outlet duct from the gall-bladder or the main duct carrying bile to the intestine.

liver. This can cause jaundice with all its accompanying complications. Stones can also cause disease of the wall of the gall-bladder and, very rarely, may give rise to cancer. A high percentage of people with gallstones, however, experience no trouble and the stones are commonly discovered as an incidental finding at autopsy.

The presence of gallstones can be compared to the tip of an iceberg as they are the visible sign of something much bigger out of sight. Gallstones develop in a relatively small proportion of people whose bile contains the wrong proportions of cholesterol and the solvent bile salts. This results in bile which is likely to give rise to the formation of stones. Almost the whole population in Western countries will have bile of a type that is more likely to give rise to gallstones than the bile of people in developing countries.

Women are much more likely to develop gallstones than men. About one woman in eight develops gallstones in most Western countries but in some communities, such as in Sweden and among the Pima Indians in the south-west of the United States, the frequency is much higher than this. The latter group, like the inhabitants of the Pacific island of .Nauru (page 28), changed their diet from a traditional type to a modern American one over a shorter period of time than did white Americans. In this way they have probably been more severely affected than the population as a whole who were subjected to far more gradual change.

79

How gallstones develop

Gallstones form when substances in solution in the bile become crystallized. The small clumps of crystals thus formed grow in size and attract other particles to them until they form tiny stones which in time grow larger.

Any increase in concentration of a substance in solution, that cna separate out as crystals, makes crystallization more likely. Decreasing the concentration will have the opposite effect. In the case of gallstones the cholesterol content of the bile is the substance that can separate out as crystals and begin the development of gallstones (facing). The most important solvent is a bile salt called chenodeoxycholate. This decreases concentration. The more cholesterol there is in the bile, the greater the tendency for gallstones to develop. The greater proportion of chenodeoxycholate there is relative to other bile ingredients the less chance of gallstones developing.

There are other factors in the development of gallstones but this is certainly the most important. Therefore anything that increases the cholesterol relative to the solvent chenodeoxycholate will tend to lead to the development of stones and anything that changes the composition of the bile in the other direction will be protective against gallstones.

There are many mechanisms that can cause gallstones but two may well relate to the refining of carbohydrate foods. Not only does fibre bind dietary cholesterol and reduce its absorption, but it also binds bile salts in the faeces so that more are eliminated in this way and less reabsorbed and returned to the liver. The first factor is believed to reduce the amount of cholesterol reaching the liver and the second increases the need for liver cholesterol to turn into bile salts. Both of these may decrease liver cholesterol.

In addition to these changes brought about by fibre in digestion, it has been shown that an increase of cereal fibre in the diet increases the production of chenodeoxycholate, which helps keep the bile cholesterol in solution. Gallstones are in fact commonly treated by prescribing chenodeoxycholate which has been taken from ox bile. This tends to dissolve gallstones but is not without side effects as well as being expensive. If it can be established that an increase in fibre-rich foods could, throughout life, maintain an adequate production of chenodeoxycholate and reduce or even prevent the formation of gallstones, then recommending dietary changes would certainly be a better

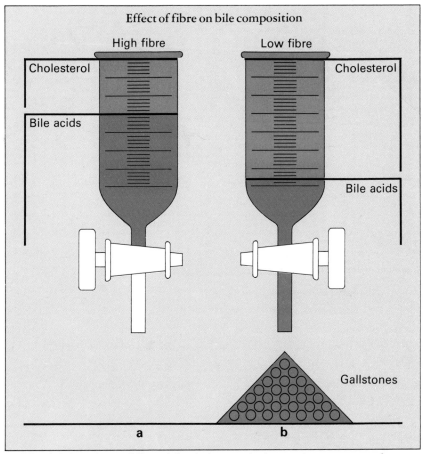

Effect of fibre on bile composition

High fibre   Low fibre

Cholesterol — Cholesterol

Bile acids — Bile acids

Gallstones

a   b

a Bile rich in solvent (bile acid) relative to cholesterol – no stones form.
b High proportion cholesterol relative to solvent (bile acid). Stones form.

approach than having to remove gallstones surgically or dissolving them with medicines after they have already developed.

Although coronary heart disease and gallstones are very different, both are associated with the production of cholesterol. In coronary heart disease it contributes to the silting-up of the arteries and in the gall-bladder it is the main ingredient of stones. Consumption of fibre-rich foods may provide some, but certainly by no means total, protection against both diseases. In the next chapter the problem of diabetes is traced to diet in a more direct way. It is worth remembering that our daily diet is one of the most potent and potentially changeable elements of our environment having far-reaching effects on health especially when continued over many years.

10 CAN DIABETES BE CONTROLLED WITHOUT DRUGS?

There are two varieties of diabetes, more correctly called diabetes mellitus (sweet urine). The common variety usually starts in middle age and is more common among people who are overweight. It can often be treated by taking tablets which lower the high blood sugar levels; other cases of diabetes are well controlled by weight reduction. A less common variety starts most often in young people and usually requires insulin injections. Only the more common variety, the adult-onset type, will be considered here.

Historical background

Diabetes was not unknown in ancient times but it was certainly rare. Indian physicians, at about the time of Christ, described diabetes. They wrote that patients passed sweet, sugary urine; this attracted flies, ants and other insects; even dogs licked the urine. About the same time Indian statues, which previously had depicted thin people, started to portray overweight middle-aged ones instead. No one reported sugary urine in Britain (as they had in Ancient Greece and Rome) until it was clearly described by Thomas Willis in 1675. He and others considered that the disease had been very rare in ancient times. This suggests that its increase has resulted from changes in environment, most probably in the food. Diabetes is more common in certain groups of people and in certain families than in others and there is undoubtedly a hereditary element. The disease does not, however, appear until specific environmental factors, in addition to the hereditary ones, have begun to operate and somehow trigger off diabetes. It seems likely that these factors are associated with diet and changes accompanying increased affluence. French physicians as late as 1870 taught that diabetes was rarely seen in the poorer hospital patients but that it was becoming increasingly common among the wealthier ones.

Who is most likely to develop diabetes?

In Western populations a fairly large proportion of people during middle age develop difficulty in utilizing carbohydrates (starch and sugar) in their diet. This difficulty is caused by a fault in insulin production in the body. Insulin is produced by the pancreas to deal with the glucose which is absorbed from the stomach and intestines. If glucose is absorbed too quickly there may be insufficient insulin to deal with all of it, and consequently the excess glucose gets into the bloodstream. This excess is known as blood sugar. If the level of blood sugar is measured several hours after the patient's last meal, it will show a rise. This is referred to as decreased carbohydrate tolerance. If the blood sugar rises too high then sugar (glucose) appears in the urine and the person may be regarded as a diabetic.

In Britain today 5 per cent of the population below the age of fifty and 15.5 per cent above that age may be considered diabetic. Diabetes is also closely associated in individuals, and in its geographical distribution, with coronary heart disease.

Available evidence suggests that diabetes became increasingly common during the last century and the early part of the present century until it reached its present frequency and then settled down to a fairly stable level. Dr H. Emerson and Dr L.D. Larimore examined the steeply rising diabetes death rate in New York City from 1888 to 1923 before the discovery of insulin. They suggested that increased consumption of sugar might be partly responsible, as had Indian physicians two thousand years before.

In Britain diabetes mortality rates fell during the food shortage in the First World War. It has been suggested that reduced sugar consumption in war-time, compared with consumption in peace-time, might account for this. Captain T.L. Cleave and Dr G.D. Campbell also traced the rise and fall of diabetic mortality from 1905 to 1947 and related this to the rise and fall of sugar consumption.

Other authorities have suggested that decreased fat intake provided a better explanation. Dr H.C. Trowell, who assisted with the writing of this book, has pointed out the possible role of dietary fibre in protecting against diabetes. He has shown that the diabetes mortality rate in Britain fell by 54 per cent between 1941 and 1953. This fall coincided with the compulsory use of high-fibre National Flour. This contained 86 per cent of the whole wheat and a greater proportion of fibre, when compared with white flour which consists of only about 72 per cent of the whole wheat. Although sugar and fat consumption in Britain during the 1950s often rose above pre-war levels, the diabetes mortality rates went on falling during all the years of the high-fibre National Bread (1941-54).

Diabetes has hardly ever been observed in any animal living in its natural environment far away from man and feeding on its usual diet. Neither has diabetes even been described in any human hunter-food gatherer. This suggests that the disease is largely the result of a man-made environment. Further evidence for this is supplied by the observation that patients suffering from diabetes, commencing in middle age, can be 'cured' and remain free of all signs of disease if they eat the traditional food of man consisting mainly of large amounts of fibre-rich starch foods. Such foods would include minimally refined cereals, such as wholemeal or rye bread, fibre-rich breakfast cereals and other fibre-rich foods which are relatively low in energy or calories. Foods such as white flour and sugar should be avoided as far as possible.

The disease has never been produced in animals by feeding them enormous amounts of sugar or fat. Nor has any human patient ever been cured of diabetes by depriving him of all sugar or of all obvious fat. Although it has been very difficult to produce diabetes in any animal, scientists have induced it in certain small rodents: sand rats, hamsters, spring mice and gerbils, in order to study its causes. All of these animals live in dry, sandy regions where food is scanty, tough and fibrous and contains little starch.

The sand rat of the Egyptian desert has been studied by scientists more than any other rodent. When this rat is offered a completely new food – a starch-rich refined wheat cereal called chow, which has much more energy (or calories) relative to its fibre than has its natural diet, it starts to eat voraciously. Energy (calorie) intake doubles and soon it becomes so fat that it can move and mate only with difficulty. (It is called *Psammonmys obesus* for this reason.)

84

Most of these rats develop diabetes and die unless given insulin. It is not necessary to add any sugar or butter to the chow to produce obesity and diabetes – their new energy-dense food is sufficient. If other sand rats in the laboratory are fed low-energy (calories) foods, such as carrots and vegetables, which contain much more fibre in proportion to their energy (calories), only a moderate amount of calories are eaten. These sand rats do not become obese or develop diabetes.

These rats have in fact undergone a similar change to that made by Western man when fibre-rich are exchanged for fibre-depleted diets and this experiment shows that such a change can result in diabetes.

As in the case of the Pima Indians, used as an example in the previous chapter, the sand rats have been subjected to a very sudden change in their diet. Similar changes in diet in Western populations usually occurred over a period of over 100 years. It is for this reason that the increased occurrence of the disease is so much more dramatic in the sand rats which have no time to adapt to their new environment.

Diabetes has been reported very rarely in any carnivore; usually, even in captivity, they remain largely flesh-eaters and refuse to eat much starch. Only about one in 800 flesh-eating cats develops diabetes but one in 200 dogs, that eat anything offered to them, develops the disease. All animals that develop diabetes, whether they are sand rats or old domestic dogs, are also overweight. Diabetes and obesity are somehow connected both in animals and in man and this suggests that there is some cause common to each disease.

Special diets to control diabetes

Many people who develop diabetes in middle age can be cured if they control their food intake so that they lose weight until it becomes normal for their height and age. If, however, they regain weight, they usually relapse. Some patients need drugs to reduce their high blood sugar levels.

It has been customary to advise diabetic patients to take little sugar and to reduce starch; this leaves a diet containing a larger proportion of fat. Recently many diabetic experts have begun to advise patients to take more starch and less fat as part of their special diet.

Some doctors have also started recommending more unrefined high-fibre starch foods (page 87). In the United States papers have been published in medical journals reporting that a diet of unrefined high-fibre starch (constituting 60 per cent of daily calorie intake with sugar reduced to 5 per cent, fat to 20 per cent and protein left at 15 per cent) caused a remission of the disease in 85 per cent of patients. These diets contain much dietary fibre – about $2\frac{1}{2}$ oz (70 g) daily.

Once the patients became free from evidence of diabetes they continued to eat a high-fibre diet. Levels of daily energy (calorie) intake were maintained as follows: starchy foods 50 per cent, fat 30 per cent, sugar 8 per cent and protein 12 per cent.

In the United States patients have not relapsed after hospital discharge, while still kept on this controlled diet for over twelve months under medical observation. The results have been confirmed at the University of Lexington, Kentucky and at several county hospitals in England. Almost all the patients that had drugs gradually removed, ceased to require them. Even those who depended on small doses of insulin often found that injections were no longer necessary. This change of diet for diabetics should of course be attempted only under medical supervision. No juvenile diabetes has yet been treated successfully using this type of diet.

It looks as if adult-onset type of diabetes, as well as being due to an inherited susceptibility, is most likely to appear among those who eat refined low-fibre carbohydrate foods. It decreases, and possibly even disappears, if the diet reverts to the traditional food of Western man. This is because increasing the proportion of high-fibre carbohydrate eaten in the daily diet has the effect of slowing down the rate of absorption of nutrients from the intestine into the body. This reduces the need for insulin production to deal with the glucose. To achieve this it is necessary to increase the proportion of our energy needs, supplied by fibre-rich starchy foods, from the present 30 to 50 per cent. Average diets in Britain or North America today contain only about $\frac{3}{4}$ oz (20 g) of dietary fibre. To increase unrefined starch to 50 per cent, fat and sugar, both containing much energy but no fibre, would have to be reduced by 10 per cent.

RIGHT: These percentages of daily energy (calorie) intake from different types of food show that the diet used so successfully in the treatment of diabetes in some centres today is similar to that eaten in Western countries when diabetes was still relatively rare and also to that eaten in countries where it is still uncommon.

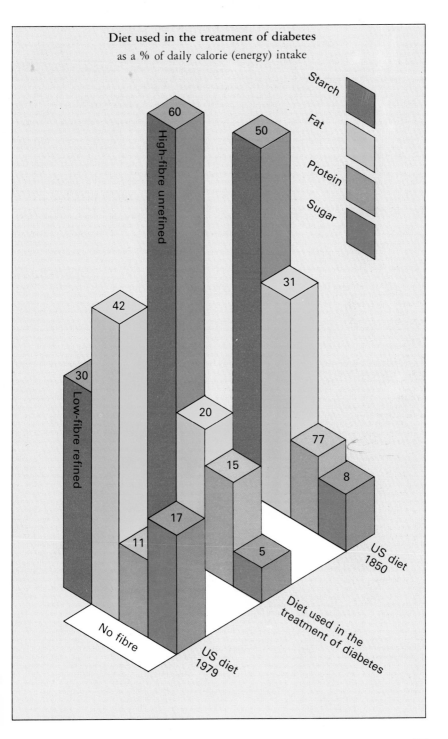

Diet used in the treatment of diabetes
as a % of daily calorie (energy) intake

Starch
Fat
Protein
Sugar

60
50
42
30
31
20
77
15
17
8
11
5

High-fibre unrefined
Low-fibre refined
No fibre

US diet 1979
US diet 1850
Diet used in the treatment of diabetes

Recent work has shown that gums, which are a constituent of certain types of fibre, increase the viscosity of the content of the small intestine, and this delays the absorption of glucose and other nutrients from the bowel into the body. The situation can be likened to watering a strip of garden. If the can has no rose the water flows out quickly and is all used up within a few yards. If, on the other hand, the water is controlled with a rose it comes out more slowly and is evenly distributed along the whole length of the garden. In like manner nutrients are absorbed quickly in the first part of the intestine – when fibre-depleted diets are eaten. They are absorbed slowly throughout the whole of the small intestine when the content has been rendered more viscid by the presence of certain gums. The former situation makes much greater demands on the insulin-secreting glands than does the latter. It is interesting that doctors who have tried these new diets sometimes add bran to the diet to get the patient off the last few units of insulin or the last tablet.

It is early days yet to assess the value of diets containing a high proportion of unrefined, fibre-rich starch foods in the treatment of mature-type diabetes. No patient already under treatment should change his own diet without medical advice and supervision. But no one can deny the potential provided by these findings nor the practical possibilities they offer.

11 THE DANGERS OF OBESITY

Why is it a problem?

Obesity means that a person weighs more than he should – for his height and age – to remain healthy and resist disease. Obesity occurs when there is an excess of fat in the body. Life insurance companies, who recognize the extra risks of obesity, insist that middle-aged candidates for life insurance must be weighed. Overweight men and women develop more diabetes and more high blood pressure than those of normal weight. Most people want to keep slim in order to be physically fit and remain attractive. One third of all British women admit that they have been trying to slim. In the United States 40 per cent of adults are overweight.

Is obesity only to do with over-eating?

One person can eat like a horse, stuffing himself with all the fattening foods, yet never gets fat. Another may eat far less, yet cannot stay slim. This does not seem fair; but then people differ in all sorts of ways. One person may have red hair and another black. One may be unable to eat strawberries while another may have trouble after eating vinegar. In a similar way people differ with regard to slimness and obesity.

Years ago most people had to do hard physical work for many hours every day. Not only did men and women walk many miles to their work, but their work also demanded much heavy exertion. Formerly women had to wash clothes, scrub floors, carry all the grocery foods from the shops and often work in the fields. Nowadays machines transport us to our jobs while other machines do all the heavy work in factories and at home. Small wonder some people get fat. We simply do not burn up the calories consumed and they are consequently stored as fat.

Appetite is influenced by our minds as well as by our physical needs. We may not need large quantities of food to provide energy but we certainly can get into the habit of eating it. We chew food or gum, eat sweets and nibble biscuits, espcially when worried or tired. We are tempted by advertisements of exciting new luscious foods. In all sorts of ways we are urged to eat and drink more and at the same time purchase machines that will save us the physical exertion needed to use up the extra calories.

Few people realize that about 10 per cent of most sweetened soft drink is composed of sugar. In its modern refined form sugar consists of calories. For a dramatic illustration of the amount of refined sugar, compared to the amount of unrefined sugar beet from which it would be extracted, see page 92. Alcoholic drinks are also fattening. Moreover, after one or two drinks, a person forgets that he was trying to slim so he eats more.

When poverty and unemployment were rife it was considered a sign of wealth to eat well and look fat; obesity was viewed as a status symbol. Fashions change, however, and people today are ashamed, rather than proud, of their expanding waistlines. Miss World and all her rivals are always slim. In this case fashion makes sense. Obese people have a higher risk of developing diseases, like coronary heart disease and diabetes, as well as looking less attractive.

Obesity: a modern disease

Undoubtedly there were some fat people in the ancient civilizations of Egypt, Assyria, Rome and Greece. They were few if one can judge from the literature and the ancient statues of those times. Even the Roman emperors in old age were seldom depicted as being grossly fat (right).

The British National Portrait Gallery shows us slim kings, queens and courtiers from the thirteenth to the middle of the seventeenth century. Charles II, in the late-seventeenth century, was the first man in the whole gallery to have a really fat tummy. Soon after this, in the reign of Queen Anne, nearly every lord and lady, even in their mid-thirties,

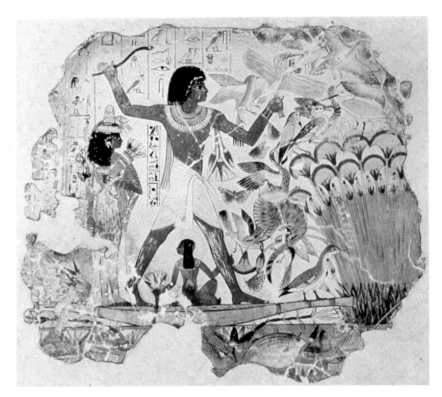

Ancient art such as this Egyptian tomb painting rarely depicted any fat people.

was definitely obese. Before that time obesity was uncommon. History books record that in the seventeenth century the British army had 40,000 men, all of whom could march well because 'not a single soldier was fat'. Few authors used the word obese before the nineteenth century. When the word was first used it simply denoted 'having eaten' and did not allude to being fat.

Just as obesity has emerged as a common condition in Western countries over the past few centuries it has more recently emerged in the less developed countries of Africa and in similar situations elsewhere in the Third World. In the 1920s doctors in East Africa reported that almost every African was slim. Even the soldiers who were liberally fed with traditional African food rarely appeared obese. In contrast urban Africans are commonly obese today and some of the overweight rulers are familiar figures on news media. When surgeons operate on the average African they find very little fat between the skin and muscle. In

91

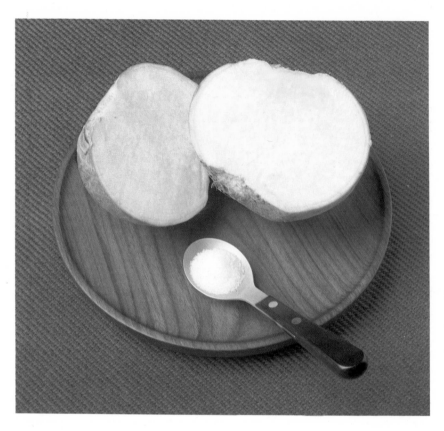

A whole sugar beet will provide just one teaspoonful of refined sugar.

people in Western countries (and Westernized Africans) there is often several inches of subcutaneous fat round the abdomen before muscle is reached.

Africans, however, even in the past knew how to make a person fat. In the 1920s, though they bought no sugar in the shops, girls were fattened to ensure good marriage prices. Girls in some tribes were encouraged to drink lots of milk and cream, both containing fat which has a high-calorie content and contributes to obesity.

Changes in eating patterns

Scientists talk about 'energy-dense' foods meaning that they contain a lot of energy in a small amount of food. In this sense both fats and sugar are 'energy-dense' foods, the former more so.

Not only are many modern Western foods 'energy-dense', and consequently tend to produce obesity, but lack of physical exercise also increases the tendency to put on weight.

Sugar often provides as much as 20 per cent of the energy consumption in modern Western diets. That is, 20 per cent of the calories eaten in a day come from sugar. Fat contributes 40 per cent of the energy (or calories) we eat. Since neither of these foods contains any fibre, 60 per cent of the energy eaten is devoid of fibre and is consequently a very concentrated source of calories. Fibre is the only component of our food that contains almost no calories.

About 200 years ago 70 per cent of the energy in the average British diet came from wheat and most of this was eaten in the form of high-fibre wholemeal bread. Sugar at that time contributed less than 4 per cent of energy. There is less knowledge of fat consumption at that time but it was certainly less than half the present levels, say up to 20 per cent of total energy in 1780.

Traditional African diets resemble, in the proportions of fat and carbohydrate, ancient British diets. Modern African diets, however, contain much more fat and sugar than previously, often with the addition of white bread. Fat and sugar contain no fibre at all and white bread only a little.

Obesity can be compared to a bank balance. A fat balance accumulates in a bank account if more money is paid in than is paid out. Similarly, obesity slowly occurs in a person if his intake of food exceeds the amount of energy used to keep his muscles moving and the various organs of his body functioning normally. The excess is stored as fat in the body. It is all a question of balance.

There must be some secret chemical messenger that detects excessive storage of fat and travels in the bloodstream to the brain where a lot of nerve cables end in what is referred to as the 'appetite centre'. This centre is apparently informed when the fat stores decrease, then in some mysterious and unknown way we get just a bit more hungry and decide to have another potato or another slice of bread and butter.

Medical science has usually given its verdict thus: obesity occurs if energy (calories) in the food exceeds energy used in working the muscles and keeping the body alive. This is not a wholly correct statement. A more accurate statement is: obesity occurs if energy (calories) *absorbed* from the food eaten exceed the energy used in the functions of the body.

High-fibre foods reduce not only the amount of energy consumed but also decrease absorption of energy by 1 to 2 per cent.

Fibre and obesity

Captain Cleave was one of the first doctors to point out that wild animals seldom get fat (except of course when they develop fat to use in winter). Neither did the average man in Europe get fat until about the eighteenth century. If an antelope gets too fat on the African grasslands a lion will catch it easily. Evolution works like that. A rabbit in Britain must remain slim or a fox will catch it. Hunter-gatherers, such as African Bushmen today, or the Australian aborigines as seen by Darwin during the nineteenth century, were always slim. A fat hunter could catch few animals; an obese food-gatherer's wife could gather few nuts and seeds.

Natural selection, in evolution, is always against obesity – unless it is an advantage to survival; some fat is necessary for seals who must store fat for they feed mostly in the short Arctic summer. Zebras also must store some fat for they get little food in the dry rainless season, but they must not get too fat or lions will catch them. Even peasant agriculturalists must not get too fat or they will be unable to engage in the hard digging and carrying necessary for their survival.

Can fibre keep you slim?

The type of obesity common in Western countries occurs when someone slowly develops an extra 14 lb (6.4 kg) of fat over fifteen years, from twenty-five until forty years old. This is 1 lb (.500 kg) per year. Food tables tell us that this can occur if only about forty extra calories are stored each day out of the daily intake of about 2000 calories. This represents only 2 per cent extra to requirements. Fibre is the only constituent in our daily diet that contains no energy (calories). If a high-fibre diet decreases energy *absorbed* from 1 to 2 per cent it seems reasonable to assume that fibre-rich food helps to keep a person slim.

Fibre helps slimness in many other ways. You have to eat wholefoods more slowly because the food needs more chewing. This means you will probably swallow more saliva which helps to fill your stomach. The fibre is bulk-forming but still contains no calories. A person tends to eat less bulky wholemeal bread than soft white bread or cake and biscuits.

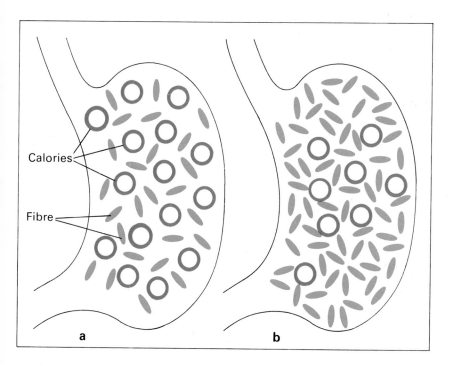

a Stomach filled with fibre-depleted food.
b Somach filled to satiety with fibre-rich food.

Bulky high-fibre foods such as wholemeal bread, potatoes and vegetables fill you up and consequently fewer calories are consumed. Sugary drinks are soon completely absorbed, so that an hour or two later you feel empty and hungry again and look round for an extra snack to eat. Fibre also retains water as discussed in earlier chapters. When adequate fibre is eaten both the small and the large intestine contain more watery material. When the bowels are full you do not feel so empty.

Fibre therefore both increases, and prolongs, feeling 'full-up' as explained in chapter five. This was demonstrated in a recently published experiment where apples were consumed in different forms. Volunteers were given equivalent amounts of apple in the form of ordinary raw apples, apple purée and apple juice (overleaf). The raw apples contained their natural skeleton of fibre; they consequently took longer to eat and satisfied hunger for a longer period of time than did apples eaten in the other two forms. The apple purée contained its fibre but it was broken

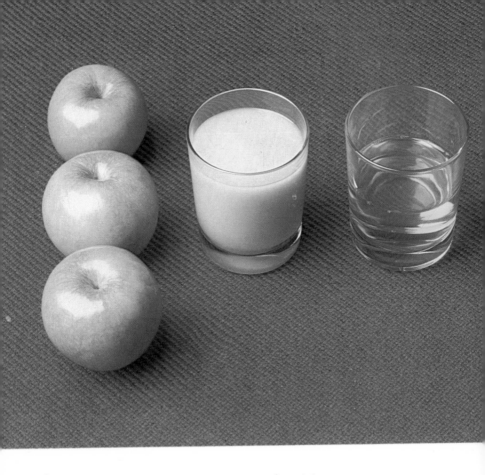

Three apples will provide this much purée or juice.

down, swallowed fairly quickly and proved less satisfying. The apple juice which contained almost no fibre was swallowed quickly and satisfied hunger least.

Are unrefined starch foods fattening?

Contrary to generally accepted opinion it has been proved that these foods are not fattening. This is because they are rich in bulky fibre. Potatoes, for example, are not fattening provided they are neither cooked nor eaten with oil or fat. Their calorie value is in fact slightly more than apples and slightly less than pears. This was shown by an experiment involving twenty-three young Irishmen. They were persuaded to eat 2 lb (about 2 kg) of potatoes, this is about ten large

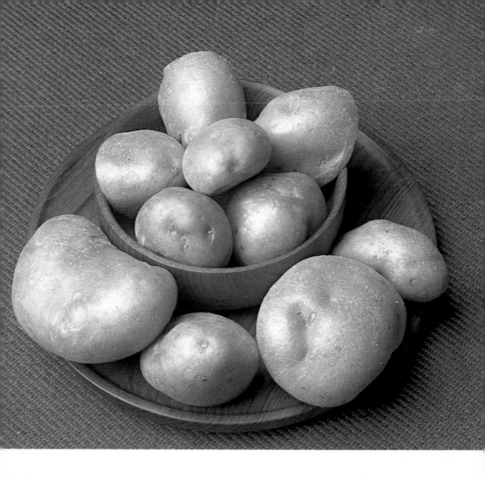

Ten large potatoes eaten daily helped men lose weight.

potatoes, every day for three months (as above). As long as they ate all the potatoes they were allowed to add as many other foods as they wanted. Actually most of the men had lost weight by the end of the three months. Eating such a large volume of potatoes fills the stomach and so prevents the consumption of other high-calorie foods.

Modern medical research is beginning to study the different response of the stomach, intestines and large bowel to high-fibre diets. It is clear already that the complicated digestive glands, such as the insulin-producing pancreas, respond differently to high-fibre diets than they do to (usual) low-fibre modern diets. Scientists believe that the former diets produce a more favourable insulin response than the latter. This may explain why high-fibre diets often help middle-aged diabetics, as described in chapter ten.

Overcoming and avoiding obesity

It is no easy thing to lose weight. If you are strong-minded you can lose several pounds, even a stone or two, over a period of several months. But if you are not careful you may gradually regain the weight and be back to square one within a couple of years. Most of us have been taught bad eating habits from childhood. We learn to prefer foods which have a low-fibre and high-energy (calorie) content — those that look so attractive in advertisements — and contain much fat and sugar. Even after successful dieting we will often gradually return to them. Such foods include ice-cream, chocolates, sweets and cakes. In addition our tastes are geared to fat taken in large amounts of butter, cream and milk and also vegetable oils, used in frying, and salad dressing. These foods should be eaten sparingly by those with a tendency to put on weight.

It is best to try to lose weight slowly over a period of six to twelve months, and then to continue indefinitely the new food habits, rather than to half-starve for a few weeks. No one can stay semi-starved for long. You do better reducing weight slowly, taking half portions of all ordinary foods that contain much fat or sugar, and eating more fish or lean meat like chicken, vegetables and fruit.

There are many books about slimming and it is impossible to write fully about it here. Two points must be made. Books on slimming give long lists of foods to avoid: sugar, butter, cream, sweets, cakes, sweetened soft drinks and alcoholic drinks. As well as being high in calories these foods contain very little or no fibre, though this is rarely mentioned. Books also give long lists of foods that may be eaten because, by themselves, they are seldom fattening. These slimming foods include vegetables, fruits, wholemeal bread, rye crispbread and so on. These foods contain much fibre, a fact that is also rarely mentioned.

It is difficult to prevent obesity in the modern world. People rightly enjoy eating. Both fat and sugar increase the palatability of foods. There are, however, many ways in which high-fibre foods, containing less fat and less sugar, can be made appetizing. Newer cookery books are beginning to emphasize the importance of high-fibre foods and it is worth trying the recipes that include them. You may find, as many others have done, that wholemeal bread and other high-fibre foods have more flavour than white bread, even though at first this may not be appreciated. In the next chapter practical suggestions will be given on how to choose the best sources of fibre from readily available foods.

12 HOW CAN WE CHANGE OUR DIET?

What changes in diet should be made to help prevent the many common ailments described in this book? The answer varies for individuals but there are certain guidelines. There are, for a start, the dietary recommendations made by the United States Senate Select Committee on Nutrition and Human Needs to improve the health of the citizens of the USA. They are recommendations from which we can all benefit (overleaf).

In addition, this chapter presents a simple guide to foods containing fibre and offers practical suggestions on how you can change your diet to increase its fibre content.

Dietary goals – The US Senate Select Committee on Nutrition and Human Needs

The accompanying diagram summarizes the conclusions of this Committee which made recommendations in 1977 on the nutritional needs of Americans. You can see that the goals, especially the first three, are in keeping with the suggestions already made in this book. The first advises a *doubling* of the proportion of energy or calories eaten by each American in his or her daily diet from starchy, carbohydrate foods, rich in fibre; it is also advised that cereal carbohydrate should have less of its fibre extracted. To double the proportion of carbohydrate foods there would need to be an increased consumption of wholemeal bread, peas, beans, lentils and root vegetables like potatoes, carrots and parsnips. The Committee advised that the energy (calorie) intake from fat should be substantially reduced overall by nearly a third and sugar consump-

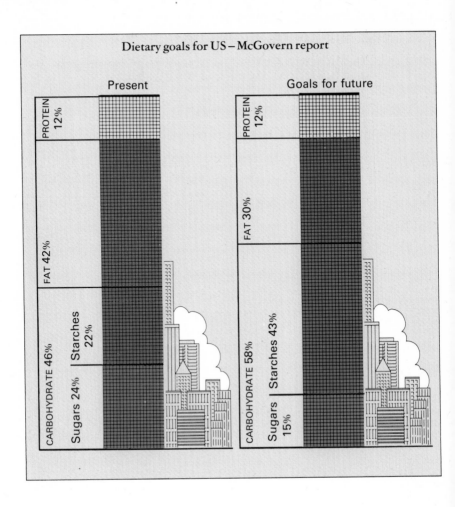

Dietary goals for US – McGovern report

tion cut by over a third. Protein levels should remain unchanged.

To achieve such a reduction of fat levels less meat and dairy products should be consumed and visible fat on meat removed before eating. Candies, sweets, pastries and cream cakes, which are rich in both sugar and fat, should be eaten sparingly.

The Committee also recommended a reduction of eggs, butter and cholesterol-rich foods. This was because of the assumed correlation between cholesterol intake and cholesterol levels in the blood. This assumption is currently still a matter of great debate among medical scientists.

The daily level of salt consumption was advised to be halved – due to its effect on high blood pressure.

Which foods have most fibre?

So which foods should you try to eat more of to increase fibre in your diet?

The accompanying table analyses the dietary-fibre content of daily foods as a percentage of their weight. The fibre content of the following types of food is given in ascending order:

Fruits and leafy vegetables – such as lettuce, cabbage and celery

Root vegetables – including tubers such as potatoes, carrots, parsnips, turnips and sweet potatoes

Legumes – including peas, beans and lentils. Nuts and dried fruits

Whole cereal – (minimally refined) – wheat, rice, corn (maize), barley, rye, millet and fibre-rich breakfast cereals

Wheat bran (miller's bran)

Try to increase the proportion of food in your daily diet from among the last three groups.

The best way to increase intake of fibre-rich food is to increase bread consumption, making sure that white bread is replaced by bread made from flour that is as near as possible to wholemeal. Although wholemeal bread has four times the amount of dietary fibre compared to white bread, its effect on bowel behaviour and content is even greater than this. Weight for weight, it is eight times more effective than white bread in treating constipation and its consequences (overleaf).

Wholemeal flour contains 100 per cent of the wheat grain after removal of the husk. White flour contains a little over 70 per cent of the grain – the remainder, containing most of the fibre and much of the mineral and vitamin content, having been removed during milling. Replacement of the minerals and vitamins removed (but not of the fibre) is compulsory by law in many countries. Starch is the main ingredient of white flour which, though deficient in crude fibre, does have a useful amount of dietary fibre, but not nearly as much as wholemeal flour.

When buying bread look for the packs labelled 'wholemeal'. Recently many bakers have tried to avert declining sales of white bread by introducing brands of 'brown' bread, sometimes with a speckling of wheat grains on the outside. The fibre content of such loaves varies

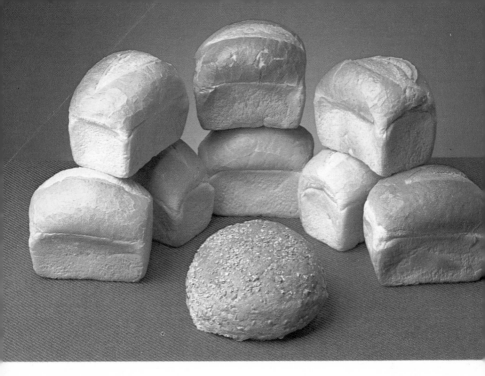

Eight white loaves would have the same effect for increasing stool output as one wholemeal.

greatly and you should ask from which type of flour they were baked.

The flour used to bake most brown breads, though less refined than white, still has much of its fibre extracted. This bread may be labelled 'wheatmeal'. The fibre content of this will be roughly halfway between wholemeal and white bread. If you buy rye bread be sure that it has been baked with unrefined rye flour. Bakers often bake so-called 'rye' bread with refined rye flour, merely adding some rye seeds to it. I know it can often be a problem for shoppers to be sure they are getting genuine wholemeal bread. Possibly only by consumer groups bringing pressure to bear for the fibre content of the flour to be shown on the wrapping can this situation be overcome.

Our ancestors ate about $1\frac{1}{4}$ lb (over 600 g) of bread, made from little-processed flour, per person per day. Current intake in Western countries is usually only about $\frac{1}{4}$ lb (120 g) of white bread. Between $\frac{1}{4}$ and $\frac{1}{2}$ lb (120-240 g) of wholemeal bread daily would be adequate to supply most of the fibre necessary to combat constipation. Fibre from other sources besides bread would also be required.

The value of bran

Another good way of meeting fibre requirements is from fibre-rich breakfast cereals. There are many varieties on the market. All those containing the word 'bran', and several others besides, are good sources of fibre.

The richest of all sources of cereal fibre is wheat bran composed of the outer layers of the wheat which are removed in the preparation of white flour (page 40). This can be bought as miller's bran. Try to get the fairly coarse flakes, rather than fine, as they are more effective. Two heaped dessertspoonfuls (tablespoons in the US) a day provide about $\frac{1}{2}$ oz (15 g) of bran containing $\frac{1}{4}$ oz (7 g) of dietary fibre. This is more than enough for most people to revolutionize beneficially their bowel behaviour.

Vegetables and fruit

Cereals and also, to a slightly less extent, peas, beans and nuts are richer in fibre than are fruits and leaf vegetables, largely because the last two consist mostly of water. Cereals are also much richer in certain constituents of fibre known as pentoses. These pentoses are the part of fibre that most increases the bulk and softness of stools. So cereals contain not only more fibre than leafy vegetables like lettuce but also far more pentoses. This means they are much more effective for increasing stool weight. Legumes, that is peas, beans and lentils, are the next best source of fibre after cereals. There is 1 oz (30 g) of dietary fibre in 9 oz (280 g) of frozen peas and a little more in the same weight of canned baked beans.

Root vegetables, including tubers like potatoes and carrots, can provide an adequate fibre intake. Considerable quantities have to be eaten, however, as illustrated. Potatoes baked in their skins have a higher fibre content, as can be seen in the table, than boiled, peeled potatoes. Although some vitamins are lost in the actual boiling of these and other vegetables, our bodies have become adjusted over innumerable generations to eating boiled food.

The main thing to remember when eating potatoes is to avoid having them fried which adds a high concentration of fat and doubles their calorie content. As mentioned earlier, potatoes are not fattening unless cooked in fat or eaten with butter or cream. In fact, the energy or calorie content per unit weight is slightly more than for apples and less than that of pears. More potatoes, though, are usually eaten at one meal. Incredible though it may seem, during the nineteenth century farm

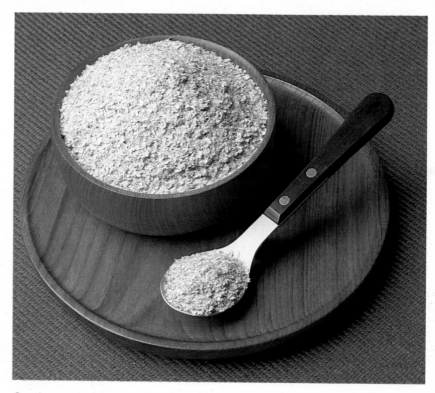

One heaped tablespoonful of bran eaten daily is usually sufficient to combat constipation.

labourers in Ireland lived on one pint of milk and ten pounds of potatoes a day. Although this diet can hardly be considered ideal, it apparently fulfilled their nutritional needs. Fresh fruit and vegetables contain fibre but they are composed largely of water. In the case of salads, for instance, it clearly would not be possible to eat anywhere near the quantity that would be required to meet our fibre requirements (right). There has been a trend to eat more salad, consisting largely of lettuce, heavily soaked in salad dressing containing fat. Professor Peter Van Soest – one of the greatest fibre experts in North America – has stated that 'salad is little more than packaged water'. Spinach does have a relatively high fibre level as you can see from the table.

An overall change in diet

Reduction in consumption of fatty foods, especially animal fats, implies a reduced intake of meat and, in particular, of red meat such as beef,

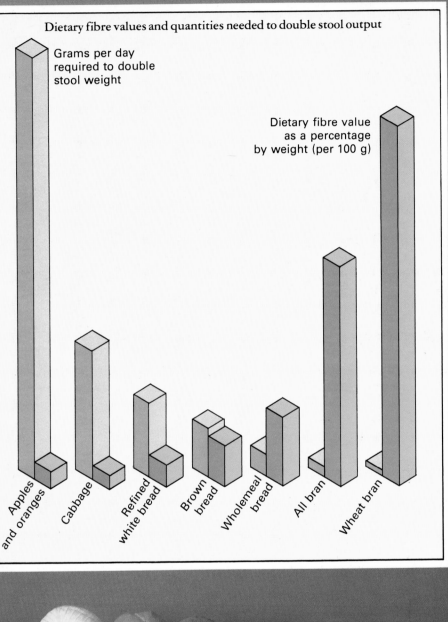

Dietary fibre values and quantities needed to double stool output

Grams per day
required to double
stool weight

Dietary fibre value
as a percentage
by weight (per 100 g)

Apples
and oranges

Cabbage

Refined
white bread

Brown
bread

Wholemeal
bread

All bran

Wheat bran

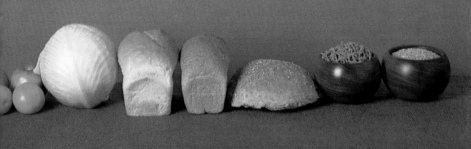

lamb and pork. Animals providing these meats have been specifically bred to increase the fat in their carcasses. Try to eat leaner meats instead of fatty ones. White meats, such as fish and poultry, have a much lower fat content, but duck and goose are rich in fat.

Consumption of refined carbohydrate foods, of which sugar is the most obvious example, should be reduced. We need to cut sugar to half or less of our present consumption of about 120 lb (50 kg) per person per year. The photograph (see page 92) gives an idea of the dramatic difference highly refined sugar has on our diet. So eat fewer sweetened foods and drink less cola and other soft drinks which all contain about 10 per cent sugar by weight. Foods composed largely of sugar and white flour should be consumed sparingly though it would be quite impractical and inacceptable to suggest that such foods should be entirely excluded from our diet. But remember that cakes, biscuits, jams, sweetened spreads, pastries, bought and home-made desserts, all contain high quantities of sugar, and often of fat, and their constituents are almost totally depleted of fibre.

Practical hints – what to eat, what to avoid

- Eat brown or preferably wholemeal bread rather than white. When you make sandwiches try to have more bread and less filling in each one.
- Substitute wholewheat flour (or near relation) for white in home-made bread, pastries, cakes, biscuits.
- Look for wholemeal pasta, such as spaghetti and macaroni, also wholewheat or bran crispbreads; brown unpolished rice (this takes longer to cook than white rice – approximately $\frac{3}{4}$ hour).
- Digestive biscuits are made from wholewheat flour.
- Choose fibre-rich breakfast cereals, many of which are described using the word 'bran'.
- Boil or bake potatoes in their skins.
- Eat nuts and dried fruits. Use lentils, beans and peas.
- Eat meat no more than once a day and, when you do, eat it sparingly. About 4 oz (120 g) is quite sufficient for an adult.
- Cut out fatty parts of meat. Leanest meats are chicken and turkey.
- White fish is less fatty than others such as mackerel, salmon, sardines, and has less calories than meat, weight for weight.

106

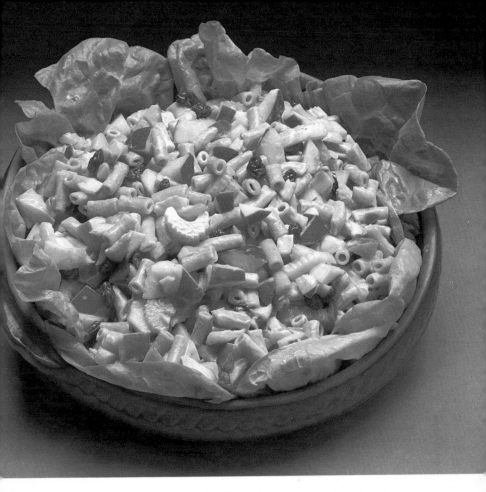

This appetizing dish was made using fibre-rich pasta produced with unrefined flour.

- Use butter sparingly. Add less cream to puddings and reduce sugar as much as possible.
- Grill instead of fry: use non-stick pans for frying with minimum fat.
- Brown sugar has little more nutritional value than white; both are termed empty calories because they provide energy but virtually nothing else.
- When possible eat fresh rather than canned fruit. The latter usually has a high sugar content.
- Drink sweetened drinks sparingly. They have a high sugar content.
- Reduce salt in diet by using sparingly in cooking, seldom adding more when eating. Smoked fish and meats have a high salt content.

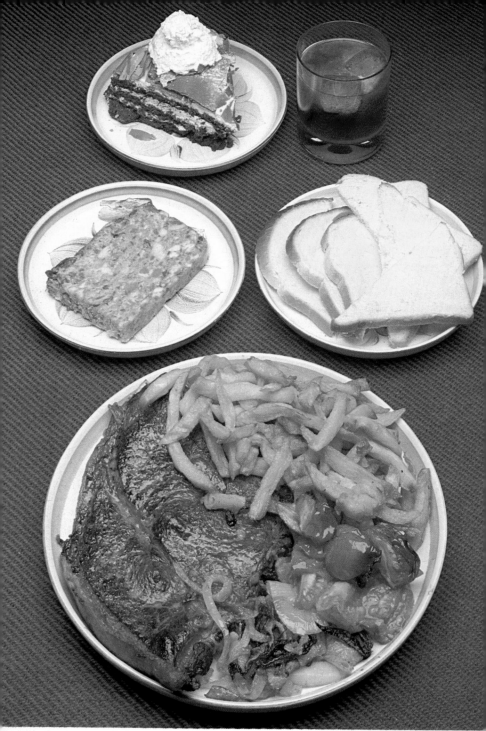

ABOVE: This meal contains minimal fibre but too much fat and sugar including the paté (high fat) and the cola drink (10% sugar).

RIGHT: Most of the food shown here is rich in fibre while containing little fat and no added sugar including the wholemeal apple pie.

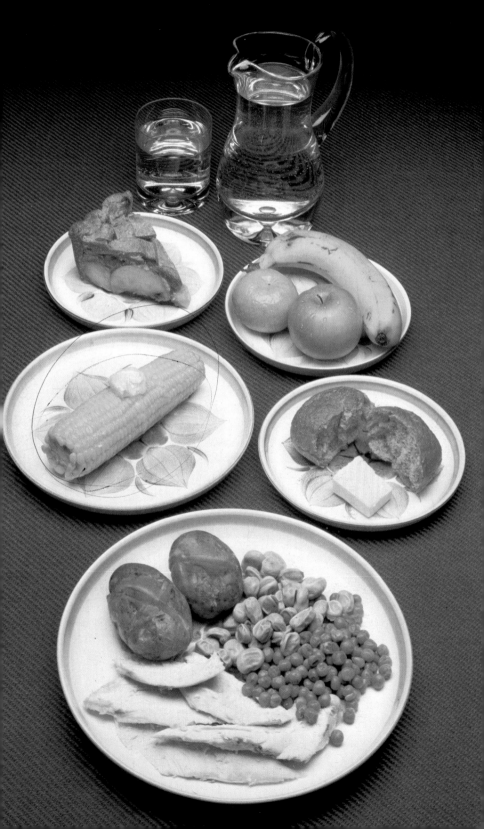

DIETARY FIBRE VALUES OF FOOD

Expressed as a percentage by weight (per 100 grams)

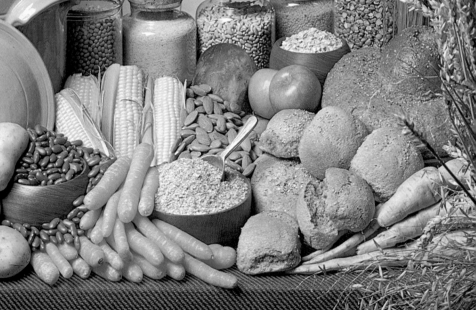

Cereals	%
Wheat bran (miller's bran)	44.0
Wholemeal flour (100% unrefined)	9.6
Brown flour (85% refined)	7.5
White flour (72% refined)	3.0
Soya flour (low fat)	14.3
Sweetcorn, canned	5.7
Corn-on-the-cob, boiled	4.7
Rice, white polished, boiled	0.8
brown, unpolished, boiled	5.5

Bread	
Wholemeal	8.5
Brown	5.1
Hovis (UK)	4.6
White	2.7

Breakfast cereals	
All Bran	26.7
Puffed Wheat	15.4
Weetabix	12.7
Shredded Wheat	12.3
Cornflakes	11.0
Muesli	7.4
Grapenuts	7.0
Sugar Puffs	6.1
Special K	5.5
Rice Krispies	4.5
Porridge	0.8

Biscuits	
Crispbread rye (Ryvita)	11.7
Digestive, plain	5.5
Wheat starch-reduced crispbread (Energen)	4.9
Shortbread	2.1

Nuts	
Almonds	14.3
Coconut, fresh	13.6
Brazil	9.0
Peanuts	8.1
Hazel	6.1

Leaf vegetables	
Spinach, boiled	6.3
Broccoli tops, boiled	2.9
Spring greens, boiled	3.8

	%
Brussel sprouts, boiled	2.9
Cabbage, boiled	1.8
Cauliflower, boiled	1.8
Celery, raw	1.8
Lettuce	1.5

Root vegetables	
Horseradish, raw	8.3
Carrots, boiled	3.0
raw	2.9
Parsnips, boiled	2.5
Beetroots, boiled	2.5
Potatoes, baked in skins (flesh only)	2.5
boiled (new)	2.0

Legumes	
Peas, frozen, boiled	12.0
Beans, haricot (whole beans), boiled	7.4
baked and canned in tomato sauce	7.3
Peas, canned	6.3
fresh, boiled	5.2
Broad beans, boiled	5.1
Lentils, split, boiled	3.7
Runner beans, boiled	3.4

Fruits	
Dates, dried	8.7
Blackberries	7.3
Raisins	6.8
Cranberries	4.2
Bananas	3.4
Pears fresh, eating	3.3
Strawberries	2.2
Plums, raw, eating	2.1
Apples	2.0
Oranges	2.0
Tomatoes, raw	1.5
Pineapple, fresh	1.2
Grapefruit	0.6

Puddings	
Apple crumble	2.5
Fruit pie	2.4
Rhubarb, stewed — no sugar	2.4
Christmas pudding	2.0
Sponge	1.2

Points about bran

As a treatment for constipation unprocessed bran has been found to be most effective, though processed bran in popular breakfast cereals is also helpful. Unprocessed bran, from health food shops and many supermarkets, can be sprinkled on stewed fruits, mixed into soups or home-made bread. When making bread add 1-2 oz (30-60 g) to 1 lb (500 g) of flour.

Start with one heaped teaspoonful a day, increasing by one heaped teaspoon after the first week. Then increase gradually as needed till at least one soft stool is passed daily, and keep to this daily amount. You may experience wind for several weeks while you are new to bran, but eventually this will disappear. It is possible to obtain bran tablets or other concentrated-fibre products. These are useful for holidays and times spent away from home when fibre-rich meals may not be available, but even for these occasions an increasing number of people carry their bran with them.

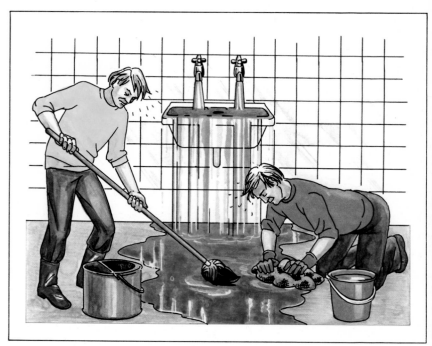

These two men are fruitlessly mopping up the overflowing water while omitting to turn off the tap or faucet.

13 NOT BY BREAD ALONE

Prevention, as we all know, is far preferable to cure. It is often more of an effort to achieve, however, because it involves changing peoples habits and attitudes.

Most modern medicine is concentrated on cure rather than prevention. It can be compared to stationing an ambulance at the foot of a cliff to pick up the casualties as men and women fall over and sustain injuries of various kinds. The efficient ambulance takes the patients to medical centres equipped with all modern facilities and staffed with highly-trained medical teams. This is important and necessary work. But how much better it would be to erect a fence around the top of the cliff to prevent people from falling off in the first place! Giving up cigarette smoking, moderation in alcohol, fastening car seat belts, and eating a prudent diet are all examples of the way we can build fences around our cliffs and so avoid many preventable diseases.

An even more telling illustration is that of a running tap filling a basin from which the overflow is flooding the floor. Two men work long hours mopping up the water, their aim and ambition in life being to keep the floor dry (left). Yet it has never occurred to them that turning off the tap would enormously reduce the need to mop the flooded floor. The running water represents the cause of disease and the flood on the floor the diseases filling hospital beds and doctors' surgeries.

A medical student learns the standard techniques of floor mopping but has minimal instruction in finding and turning off running taps or, in other words, discovering the cause of, and eradicating, disease. Industrial enterprises provide the best mops man's ingenuity can devise

113

in the form of pharmaceutical preparations, surgical appliances and laboratory technology. For all of these we must be grateful, but let them not blind us to the need to search out and wipe out causes of disease at their source.

The analogy is plain. There is, and always will be, a flood on the floor, the presence of disease in the world, which must be dealt with by the best means possible. But how much better it would be to turn off the tap as well as mopping the floor, rather than ignoring the former while concentrating on the latter.

You could say, in the face of the ideas presented in this book, that we do not yet have sufficient proof concerning the turning off of this particular tap – fibre-depleted diets. But to use another example, if a man has fallen into the water and there is a lifebelt at hand you throw it to him. You would hardly ponder whether it is the right size, the correct shape or specific gravity while the man meanwhile drowns! The testing can be done subsequently so as to improve rescue arrangements for future needs. There is still much testing to be done regarding diet but meanwhile we do have sufficient knowledge on which we can act and also sufficient knowledge to say that, if Third-World communities adopt our kind of diet, they do so at their peril.

Beyond biological reckoning

It might well be argued – and I fully agree – that the welfare of individuals is only partially ensured by caring for their biological needs. Were a human being no more than a chemical factory, or even a purely biological creature, the adequate meeting of bodily needs alone would provide satisfaction and fulfilment, yet it is patently obvious that this is far from the case. I have endeavoured to show in this book that, from a dietary point of view, we have concentrated on the content of plant cells, the nutrients they contain and ignored the carton, the cell wall, the indigestible fibre. It is all too easy when dealing with patients to concentrate so much on the carton, man's biological body, that we ignore the content, man himself as a person. Lord Tennyson wrote 'I am not my skeleton and consequently I am not greatly concerned where my skeleton came from.' Some 5000 years before Tennyson it was written in the book of Deuteronomy 8: 5:3 that 'Man cannot live by bread alone', bread referring not only to food, an essential requirement for life, as discussed in this book, but representing all the needs of our biological natures. The quote continues 'but by every word that God utters', implying that man is something more than a merely biological creature.

In recent years there has been an increasing appreciation of the essential inter-relationship between mind and body in the maintenance of health. The Greeks used the word 'soma' to denote the body and 'psyche' to describe the mind. The term psychosomatic disease implies illness explicable in part by purely physical changes but in which other factors such as anxiety, insecurity or the tensions of a stressful relationship also play a part. Many doctors widen this concept even further to include the component of man's nature for which the Greeks used the word 'pneuma', referring to man's true self or spirit, that additional dimension which would seem to differentiate man from all other animals.

A book on the relationship between food and health must inevitably emphasize biological or body disease almost to the exclusion of other aspects of well-being. I am anxious that this should in no way detract from the truth that man is an entity comprising body, mind and spirit, an order of priorities which should be reversed in conformity with Tennyson's comment referred to above, or with St Paul's prayer for his Thessalonian friends that they be kept in spirit, mind and body (I Thessalonians 5: 5:23).

The basic concept of health is that of wholeness. This involves every component of man's being and also inter-relationships with one another. We have in our own hands the means to improve the nourishment, and consequently the health and fulfilment, of all three components of our nature. In respect of the purely biological there is far too great a tendency to resort to drugs rather than recognizing and avoiding the causes of disease. I hope this book will help to overcome this tendency.

ACKNOWLEDGEMENTS

I want to thank my wife Olive, her support and help have been invaluable not least on the many occasions when my work has taken me away from my happy home.

I am greatly indebted to Dr Hugh Trowell, former Senior Consultant Surgeon Physician at Makerere University Teaching Hospital, Kampala, Uganda. He helped write the sections on coronary heart disease, diabetes and obesity. He also assisted with research and checking.

I acknowledge with gratitude the help I have so generously received from literally hundreds of doctors, the majority serving in mission hospitals in Africa and Asia. In spite of perpetual overwork they have always been prepared to take on even more by collecting facts for me which, when strung together like beads on a string, contributed greatly to the formation of the ideas presented in this book.

I would also like to thank Surgeon Captain T.L. Cleave, formerly of the British Navy, who first introduced me to the concept that many of our characteristically Western diseases might be largely the result of the food we eat.

My warmest thanks go to Mrs Sheila King for secretarial and other assistance. And finally I am deeply grateful for the unstinting assistance and helpful advice given by my publisher, Martin Dunitz.

The Publishers would like to thank:
Arthur Guinness Son & Co. Ltd, London, for permission to reproduce
the photograph used for the frontispiece; ICI for permission to reproduce the two photographs by Lennart Nilsson of coronary arteries on
page 74; the photograph on page 91 reproduced by courtesy of the
Trustees of the British Museum; the photograph of a Waldorf Salad on
page 107 was supplied by courtesy of Pasta Foods Limited and prepared
using their *Record* unrefined pasta; Her Majesty's Stationery Office,
London, for permission to reproduce the information contained in the
table on pages 110–111 and derived from McCance and Widdowson's
The Composition of Foods, fourth revised edition by A.A. Paul and
D.A.T. Southgate published in 1978. The figure for brown,
unpolished rice given on page 110 was supplied by Dr Southgate
personally and based on one test. The figure for soya flour was derived
from other sources.

REFERENCES AND SELECT BIBLIOGRAPHY

General

Burkitt, D.P., *Brit. Med. Jour.*, vol. 1, p. 274, 1973.

Burkitt, D.P., *Lancet*, vol. 2, p. 1237, 1970.

Cleave, T.L., *The Saccharine Disease*, John Wright, Bristol, 1974.

Stanway, A., *Taking the Rough with the Smooth*, Pan Books, London and Sydney, 1976.

Trowell, H.C., *Amer. Jour. of Clin. Nutr.*, vol. 29, p. 417, 1976.

Diverticular Disease

Painter, N.S., *Annals of Royal College of Surgeons of England*, 34, p. 98, 1964.

Painter, N.S., *Diverticular Disease of the Colon*, Heinemann Medical Books, London, 1975.

Painter, N.S., and Burkitt, D.P., *Brit. Med. Jour.*, vol. 2, p. 450, 1971.

Appendicitis

Burkitt, D.P., in *Refined Carbohdyrate Foods and Disease*, eds. D.P. Burkitt and H.C. Trowell, p. 87, Academic Press, London and New York, 1975.

Short, A.R., *Brit. Jour. of Surg.*, vol. 8, p. 171, 1920.

Walker, A.R.P., Walker, B.F., Richardson, B.D. and Woodford, A., *Postgraduate Med. Jour.*, vol. 49, p. 24, 1973.

Hiatus hernia

Burkitt, D.P. in *Refined Carbohydrate Foods and Disease*, eds. D.P. Burkitt and H.C. Trowell, p. 161, Academic Press, London and New York, 1975.

Varicose veins

Adams, J.C., *Acta. Chir. Scand.*, vol. 99, p. 133, 1950.

Burkitt, D.P., *Archives of Surgery*, vol. 3, p. 1237, 1976.

Cleave, T.L., *On the Causation of Varicose Veins*, John Wright, Bristol, 1960.

Folse, R., *Surgery*, vol, 68, p. 974, 1970.

Haemorrhoids

Burkitt, D.P., and Graham-Stewart, C.W., *Postgraduate Med. Jour.*, vol. 51, p. 631, 1975.

Thomson, W.H.F., *Brit. Jour. of Surg.*, vol. 62, p. 542, 1975.

Colon cancer

Burkitt, D.P., *Cancer*, vol. 28, p. 3, 1971.

Hill, M.S., *et. al.*, *Lancet*, vol. 1, p. 95, 1971.

McLennan, R., *Lancet*, vol. 2, p. 207, 1977.

Walker, A.R.P., *Amer. Jour. of Clin. Nutr.*, vol. 29, p. 1417, 1977.

Wynder, E.L. and Reddy, B.S., *Cancer*, vol. 2, p. 111, 1974.

Coronary heart disease

Kritchevsky, O., *Amer. Jour. of Clin. Nutr.*, supplement vol. 10, p. S65, 1978.

Morris, J.N., Marr, J.W. and Clayton, D.G., *Brit. Med. Jour.*, vol. 2, p. 1307, 1977.

Trowell, H.C., *Amer. Jour. of Clin. Nutr.*, vol. 25, p. 926, 1972.

Trowell, H.C., in *Refined Carbohydrate Foods and Disease*, eds. D.P. Burkitt and H.C. Trowell, p. 195, Academic Press, London and New York, 1975.

Trowell, H.C., and Burkitt, D.P., *Artery*, vol. 3, p. 107, 1977.

Walker, A.R.P., *South African Med. Jour.*, March 1977, pp. 1-9.

Gallstones

Brett, M. and Barker, D.J.P., *International Jour. of Epidemiology*, vol. 5, p. 335, 1977.

Burkitt, D.P., and Tunstall, M., *Jour. of Tropical Medicine & Hygiene*, vol. 78, p. 140, 1975.

Heaton, K.W., in *Refined Carbohydrate Foods and Disease*, eds. D.P. Burkitt and H.C. Trowell, p. 173, Academic Press, London and New York, 1975.

Heaton, K.W., *World Medicine*, 12 July, 1978, p. 21

Diabetes

Anderson, J.W., *Amer. Jour. of Clin. Nutr.*, vol. 29, p. 895, 1976.

Heaton, K.W., Huber, G.B., Murphy, D. and Burroughs, L.F., *Lancet*, vol. 3, p. 697, 1977.

Jenkins, D.J.A., *et. al., Brit. Med. Jour.*, vol. 1, p. 1392, 1978.

Jenkins, D.J.A., *et al., Lancet*, vol. 3, p 797, 1977.

Trowell, H.C., *Diabetes*, vol. 24, p. 762, 1975.

Obesity

Heaton, K.W., *Nutrition*, vol. 27, p. 170, 1973.

Heaton, K.W., *Lancet*, vol. 2, p. 1418, 1973.

Heaton, K.W., ed., *Kellogg Nutrition Symposium — Dietary Fibre*, p. 141, Newman Publishing Co., London, 1977.

Trowell, H.C., *Plant Foods for Man*, vol. 1, p. 157, 1974.

Trowell, H.C., in *Refined Carbohydrate Foods and Disease*, eds. D.P. Burkitt and H.C. Trowell, p. 227, Academic Press, London and New York, 1975.

INDEX

intestine, large 9-10, 26, 41-5, 53, 56, 66-71, 78, 95, 97
intestine, small (gut) 9-10, 32, 41-5, 50-52, 67, 70, 71, 88, 95, 97
see also bowel
iron 39

jam 106
jaundice 78

lamb 106
Larrimore, Dr L.D. 83
laxatives 45, 46
legislation, food 15, 99
legumes 38, 39, 48, 101, 103, *110-11*
lentils 99, 101, 103, 106
lettuce 101, 103, 104
lignin 40
liver 41, *42*, 78, 80

macaroni 106
mackerel 106
maize 70
margarine 9
McGovern Committee 78
meat 9, 69, 98, 100, 104-6, 107
milk 92, 98, 104
millet 70, 101
minerals 9, 101
Mulcahy, Dr Risteárd 78

nuts 9, 40, 101, 103, 106, *110-11*

oatmeal 37
obesity 29, 76-7, 85, 89-98

oesophagus: *see* gullet
oils 9, 36, 40, 96, 98
Osler, Sir William 75

pancreas *42*, 43, 83, 97
parsnips 38, 99, 101
pasta 106, *107*
pastries 100, 106
pears 96, 103
peas 38, 39, 48, 99, 101, 103, 106
pectin 40
pentoses 40, 103
peristalsis 43
piles 10, 12, 27-8, *29*, 56, 64-5
polyps 66
polysaccharides 40
pork 106
potatoes 9, 34, 36, 38, 48, 95, 96-7, 99, 101, 103-4, 106
poultry 106
protein 9, 34, 35-6, 39, 41, 69, 70-71, 86, 87, 100
puddings 107, *110-11*

rectum 41, *42*, 43, 56-7, 66
Rendle-Short, Professor 53
rice 36, 37, 70, 101, 106, *110-11*
roughage: *see* fibre
rye 101, 102
rye crispbread 37, 98

saccharine 12
salad dressings 98, 104
salads 104
salmon 106
salt 76, 78, 100, 107
sardines 106